THE REALITY MANIFESTO

An A to Z anti-exploitation guide for social media, mental health & body image

Leanne Maskell
Illustrations by Eleanor Loseby

Acknowledgements

This book was inspired by the child who had her childhood stolen by being treated like a product, including by herself. The girl who lost connection with her body because she started using it as a tool to survive. She believed her worth could be measured and controlled by numbers, growing up trying to achieve the filtered version of herself that was constantly drummed in as being 'better' than who she was in reality.

The girl grew into an adolescent who didn't know how to live a life that wasn't based on social media. She very nearly died as a result, but survived to tell this story. She grew into a woman who understood that the things that happened to her were not her fault: they were a product of her environment.

That girl is me. I wrote this book because I see the same experiences I had imposed on entire generations of young people, along with impossible standards that simply don't exist. Many are not as fortunate as I was to have survived. Molly Russell took her own life age 14 after looking at self-harm posts on Instagram, and Frankie Thomas took her own life age 15 after looking at suicide methods online at school.

This book is for every single person that resonates with this. It's a beacon of hope, calling for change, and a reminder that **it's not your fault.**

Table of Contents

Foreword

You don't know me, but this is likely to be a familiar story...I am the mother of three teenage girls. From the beginning, I've done my, far from perfect, best and instinctively nurtured them and protected them from harm. I used to smile when I was told not to use the TV as a babysitter, as I popped them in front of CBeebies to get on with all the things I couldn't do, with a small child claiming my attention. I'd watch them play in the sandpit while chatting with other carers about the joys and despairs of life with tiny children. And I continued to watch over them and remained alert; and was wary when I saw the smart screens and social media 'take-over.' I worried when I saw the ever increasing numbers of prams being pushed by people who had eyes fixed on their devices and the increasingly younger children, even babies, who started to be given their own. As a training psychologist, but, most importantly a parent, I'd had it drummed into me how important it was, for children's healthy development, for us to be 'with' them in mind and body.

We held off giving our girls mobiles until 13, and 14 with my youngest who we knew would find it harder (she'd recently been diagnosed with ADHD). And now, well let's say my home is, more often than not, a battleground, and not around the things I'd expected and was preparing for. **The onslaught of a social media/digital world is claiming my children's attention, and so their lives.** Where to begin? The screen-time averages (don't ask!), the impact on grades, the subverting of all controls I try, the streaming of content which you know you would never normally allow your child to view if you had any idea what they were up to. But what I am truly horrified by is the impact on mental health. The levels of mental distress and disorders that flood our young people's lives cannot be normal. And I am also shocked by the number of people, many who I love and trust, telling me 'it's no worse than it used to be.' I hear from the Headmistress of a prestigious girls' school how it's the way it's being manifested that's different not the extent - 'self harm is the new eating disorder'. Or how self-harm is the new 'sad' - really! Really?! How can we be normalising this!? Are we so overwhelmed and in denial? I think we are. And we need to do something about it now.

The relief when I met Leanne, about a year ago, and poured out my worries about this. She was someone who, sadly through her own experiences, understood this and she had such insight into the damage being done. Her passion and desire to help gives me real hope she can make a positive difference by raising awareness for this and getting things done to help. I pray she can bridge the 'generation' gap I feel, and sense of powerlessness to protect my children, and myself, from forces I do not understand. The algorithms, the 'super-smart,' faceless, conglomerates who are hell bent on bleeding us dry of our 'data' and claiming our time.

Please understand, I do not believe all social media is the enemy, screens are not the enemy, but we have to know more about how we are being impacted and for what ends. Think back to the tobacco industry and how long it took to regulate this and to inform people how it was literally killing them! So we could then, at least, as informed adults, make a choice (addiction aside) about what we did. But don't we have a duty of care to protect those who are vulnerable, our children, as their parents and as a society? Would we ever leave our children in a room, intentionally, with anything we thought could harm them?

Maybe a good current analogy, although it perhaps doesn't go far enough, should be with food. Would we allow our children to sit in a room and ply themselves with junk food without even knowing what was in it, what it was doing to them, how addictive it was, what it would prevent them from doing? What about those who had diabetes or other health concerns which would make it life-threatening for them?

Do the companies who sell it to them have our children's interests at the heart of their business models?

There is a battle to be fought here, as what we need; transparency, integrity and a right to choose, are not going to be given to us unless we fight for it. There are forces at work who do not care about us, or our children, except as an opportunity to gain power or money or both. We should not be ignorant of this and if we stand back and do nothing then we are allowing this to happen. Thank you, Leanne for everything you are doing and for rallying us together to make the difference we have to make.

By Clare Harding

Introduction

Imagine this: you're a child, and it's the weekend. You wake up, and the first thing you do it reach for your phone. You check your social media feeds before anything else, feeling deflated at not having had 'much' engagement on your posts overnight. You flick from app to app, refreshing the pages for new notifications, settling on the content you're shown instead.

You spend an hour scrolling through posts of impossibly beautiful people, luxury beaches, and what hundreds of people spent their Friday night doing. You're shown 'what I eat in a day' by your favourite influencer, and feel excited at the possibility of looking like her, though her 5-second diet seems like it might be difficult at first. You see your friends' comments on each other's posts and feel scared that you've been left out. You worry about needing to post something to stay relevant.

So, you get out of bed and spend hours doing your make up from a video tutorial and picking an outfit that you haven't been 'seen' wearing before online. Another hour passes. You take selfies for another hour, getting frustrated at everything about your life and yourself for not looking 'good' in any of the photos. You swipe left onto the filters, and breathe. You finally look 'okay' – like your post might be safe from comments telling you how ugly you are.

You flick through the different filters, trying out different jawlines, noses, lips, eye colours, hair colours, eye sizes, bright white teeth, and skin tones for another hour. You finally settle on a filter called 'VS Model Perfect Face', and feel like you might even look 'good' now. You post it online, and anxiously swipe the page, hoping for notifications.

You distract yourself by liking and commenting on other peoples' posts, comparing yours to theirs, beating yourself up for not having a better background, or more followers. You decide to put your phone down, because you're getting so worked up. You catch sight of yourself in the mirror, and burst into tears, wondering why you can't look like the filtered version of yourself. You pick your phone back up and go onto profiles that explain plastic surgery in detail, feeling slightly hopeful at the beautiful, happy people that talk about how much better they feel after having surgery.

You notice that notifications have flooded in on your post, mostly from friends saying how incredible you look. You feel better for a split second, because you've found a way of looking like that in real life too, but anxious about how you'll convince your parents to let you have cosmetic surgery at 13. You feel trapped by not wanting anybody to see you as you 'really' are, in comparison to this filtered version of yourself, until that happens.

You decide that until you're 18, you can at least work on being thin. Before you know it, you're watching videos explaining how to starve yourself and hold off hunger pangs. You receive a message from a new follower asking if you want to join their 'thinspiration community'. On this community, you instantly feel validated: people are being nice to you, they're commenting on your posts, they're telling you how to be happy, by not eating. They seem to understand where you're coming from.

Before you know it, your parent is in your room, demanding to know why you haven't come downstairs for lunch. You tell them to go away, deeply entrenched in your virtual world.

Why I'm writing this book

I've been various forms of that child throughout my life, starting with being a model at the age of 13 and appearing in Vogue. I've compared myself to filtered versions of myself since I can remember and know how much pointless misery this causes. I've been trapped in the addictive cycle of seeking external validation from unhealthy places, like model agents who were pressuring me to lose weight, but I couldn't quit.

I reached the end of the rainbow – having lots of followers on social media, shooting an endless stream of 'perfect' content from professional photoshoots, lived in beautiful places, and seemed to have everything that social media holds up as the 'ideal' standards. However, in reality, this life made me so unhappy I became suicidal.

Fortunately, I was able to get help, and now live a much happier, more balanced life. I was diagnosed with Attention Deficit Hyperactivity Disorder (ADHD) when I was 25, which helped me to understand why I became so addicted to the world of social media.

However, especially through working as a Coach, I can see *everybody* is having the same experiences of objectifying themselves in this way, regardless of whether they're a fashion model or have ADHD, and especially young people.

I speak to parents daily who are in despair at how their children seem to be existing through screens, how their childhood is being stolen from them by the 5th limb they have, and how no matter how hard they try, they cannot break through. Every day, young people tell me about the pressures they feel from society, how they can't concentrate on anything longer than a few songs, and how it feels easier to numb their feelings through social media rather than exist in the 'real world'.

I've had the experience of growing up with my identity splintered and objectified online as a fashion model, appearing in women's fashion magazines every month from the age of 13. I was obsessed with posting pictures of myself on social media, growing my 'following' (even if that meant buying followers), and attached my self-worth to how many likes I had that day. Eventually, I deleted my entire account – and freed myself from this invisible mental prison. This book is to help you break free too, without necessarily having to delete your accounts.

Through studying law, I learned how exploitation worked in the fashion industry, and published best-seller 'the Model Manifesto', which helped prompt the Government take real action. Having worked in mental health law during the pandemic alongside the Government, I've seen how these issues have been amplified by social media to create a global mental health crisis impacting us all.

I hope this book will give you practical, useful advice on using social media instead of being used by it and prompt the Government to take urgent action to address the dangers posed by the addictive nature of these platforms. Any laws relating to social media must address the practical reality of what is making harmful content so popular: the algorithms.

It's not our fault we're being exploited by technology, but it is our choice to understand how this is happening, to empower ourselves, and call for action. If it was illegal for social media companies to profit from our attention via targeted advertising, we would be the customers, instead of the products.

I wrote this book because I felt I had a moral obligation to do so. I wrote it to give hope, empowerment, and choice. To give you the power of deciding what kind of life you want to live, instead of having it dictated to you by an algorithm.

Trigger warning

This book talks about everything that's available online. I share my own experiences in suffering serious mental health challenges, from eating disorders to self-harm, and planning to take my own life. I also talk about pornography, sex, violence, depression, anxiety, cosmetic surgery – basically anything that can be found on the internet.

These topics might be disturbing to read about, but I cover them because these conversations need to be had. We need to recognise that these issues exist, otherwise this silence traps us, and the people we care about, into vulnerable circumstances where exploitation can happen. Knowledge is power.

However, I am a white, privileged female. Writing this book has been incredibly difficult, and I am sure you'll find mistakes throughout, but as in 'P is for Perfection', perfect doesn't exist! Please know that I do not mean to offend anyone, and feel free to drop me a message if you've got any suggestions on hello@leannemaskell.com.

If any of the topics in this book upset you to the point you need professional support such as from a doctor, please seek it out.

If you do one thing after reading this book, please sign my petition calling for social media companies profiting from our attention to be properly regulated. Your voice matters.

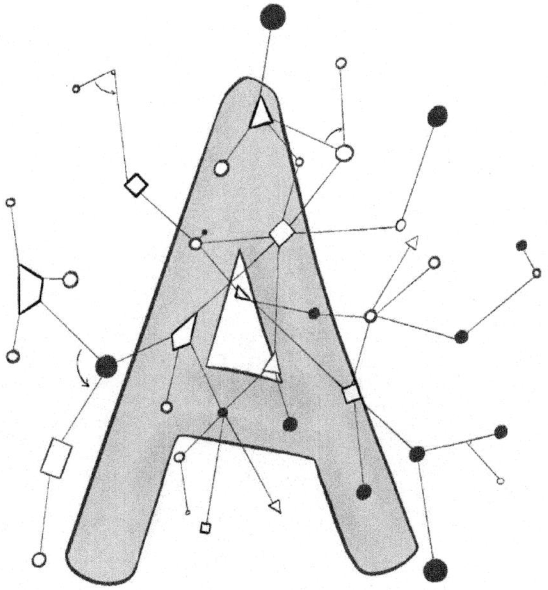

is for Algorithms

A is for Algorithms

Did you know?

- Researchers coined the term 'Variable Attention Stimulus Trait' for people experiencing symptoms of ADHD induced by the demands of modern life, which has trained us to go faster and faster, requiring constant stimulation, as most of us can go no more than a few minutes without looking at a screen.[1]

I believe social media platforms should come with similar warnings to those on cigarette packets: 'WARNING, SOCIAL MEDIA IS HIGHLY ADDICTIVE AND CAN DAMAGE YOUR HEALTH'. Teams of the best behavioural scientists and design engineers *in the entire world* have devised ways to make you as addicted as possible to these apps, because your attention is worth billions.

Just like the hidden sugar and chemicals that keep us hooked to junk food, algorithms are the invisible handcuffs keeping us chained to our phones. Though it's easy to believe it's your responsibility to manage your consumption of technology, **it's not your fault** that you're being manipulated in ways far beyond your control, making this feel impossible.

It's unfair to pit countless teams of top behavioural engineers, billions of pounds, and invisible technology against people who don't even understand what's happening to them, who ultimately, blame themselves. This is especially so for young people literally growing up on these platforms, who've maybe even had their *birth* announced on Facebook, and can't imagine a reality without social media

---

[1] Edward Hallowell and John Ratey, 'ADHD 2.0', Penguin Random House, 2021, page 15

existing. As they've only known this world, they may believe that they should be able to control it.

Have you ever wondered how platforms such as Instagram, Facebook, Snapchat, Google and TikTok are free to use, but make *billions* of pounds in revenue – some more than the income of entire countries? It's because you're not the customer, but the product, and you're being tracked, monitored, and studied by technological processes called algorithms that don't have morals, but orders.

These orders generally equate to keeping you 'engaging' with a platform for as long as possible, or on in other words, addicted. The more we use these apps, the better they become at personalizing content to us. For example, a leaked internal document exposed how TikTok's recommendation system focused on *retention* (whether a user returns to a certain kind of content), and *time spent* (how much time a user spends watching a certain kind of content).

It can predict which videos are likely to keep a person engaged by tracking their activity, such as likes and comments, literally testing out different types of content on a user to measure their engagement levels and understand them. Every millisecond of behaviour is tracked to train the algorithm on what uniquely tailored content will keep that individual using the platform instead of doing other things they want to do.

If we spend more time looking at a photo of cats than of dogs, the algorithm shows us more content relating to cats. It's a feedback loop - we're engaging with the algorithm, training it on what we're interested in, and it shows us more. This enables it to make spookily accurate predictions about our behaviour, which are sold to companies that want to influence us, as in 'M is for Money'. Social media is just the middleman, taking a huge cut of the profits.

Any platform that profits from our attention uses these algorithms to keep us addicted, and they're changing constantly, as we give them more data to work with. For example, Instagram previously showed content in a chronological order of posting, but this was changed in 2015 to prioritize 'engagement'. As in 'H is for Health', algorithms don't know the difference between healthy and unhealthy – they're simply programmed to use our curiosity and insecurity to entice us into staying for longer, at any cost.

Engagement

Engagement doesn't mean the same as enjoyment – it simply means using. As a result, our most fundamental vulnerabilities to survive and evolve are exploited by the targeting of a neurotransmitter in our brains called dopamine, which can be extremely powerful in motivating us to act. It's ignited by the thrill of uncertainty and anticipation, such as the desperation of a child wanting to open their presents on Christmas morning. It trains us to prioritize searching for potential signs of danger, seeking out updates such as changes in the weather, or liking sugary tastes so we can get energy highs until our next meal.

These evolutionary tendencies haven't caught up with the modern world, where we have easy access to non-stop sugar, news, and mental stimulation, but without the dangers of needing to fight for our survival. Every time a notification pops up, it's triggering this dopamine reward pathway. Human beings aren't designed to have dopamine spikes hundreds of times per day, which can put us into a near-constant 'fight or flight' mode of stress and anxiety, worrying about what we're missing out on.

The result is an inability to relax – ever. If your brain believes we're in constant danger, it'll keep us looking out for the next update or message, hoping this'll keep us safe, whilst keeping us addicted to the cause of our problems. Unsurprisingly, it's very difficult to concentrate on anything when we're in this state, causing a deficit of our ability to pay attention, combined with a disordered state of mental or physical hyperactivity.

In China, the laws state that there must be a 5-second gap for children after they have seen a certain number of videos on their version of TikTok, only being allowed 40 minutes of use per day in total.[2] This is pretty fascinating given that TikTok is Chinese!

ADHD / VAST

'Variable Attention Stimulus Trait' has been referred to as environmentally-induced behaviours resulting from our modern world. Researchers have commented how this change has been underappreciated, as we're experiencing it as it happens, like frogs in cold water that's slowly warmed up without the frogs trying to jump out, until they're boiled.[3]

There's no physical test to determine whether a person has ADHD or not, and no clinical recognition of VAST. Symptoms can include being disorganised to the point of chaos, irrationality, a sense of 'now or not now' as time, an inability to do things in their best interest, extremely bored by reality to the point of getting in trouble, self-sabotage, speaking without thinking, difficulties taking orders or working with others, challenges organising and acting on ideas, easily distracted, impulsive, poor short term memory, impatience, insecure, and more. These are on a spectrum, and positives can include being passionate, being able to get a lot done in a short amount of time, creativity, curiosity, energetic, tenacious, 'hyper-focus', and more.

However, this is not a neurodevelopmental condition – it's environmentally induced from the modern world. Whereas many parents would've been excited over a once-yearly trip to the cinema whilst growing up, today kids can easily sit in front of of a television, whilst being on a laptop *and* scrolling on their phones. Apps like

---

[2] Adam Smith, 'TikTok in China gets 40-minute limit for kids under new regulations', *the Independent*, 20 September 2021, accessed 20 February 2022. www.independent.co.uk/life-style/gadgets-and-tech/tiktok-douyin-china-40-minutes-limit-b1923255.html

[3] Edward Hallowell and John Ratey, 'ADHD 2.0', Penguin Random House, 2021, page 15

TikTok show a constant stream of highly stimulating videos of only a few seconds long, hooking our brains onto processing content this quickly. Algorithms cause us to experience repeated dopamine highs, leaving us on a constant search for the next thing.

It takes the average person over 23 minutes to get back to what they were doing after being interrupted. Phones can be like video games for our brains, popping up with endless different distractions, fueling habits of 'picking up' our phone to check for new messages, which become ingrained into our brains, even when we're talking to other people.

Whereas we might have once been able to control the distractions in our life, for example by getting a drink when television adverts came on every 15 minutes, now, they bombard us 24 hours per day in ways that are far less obvious, such as 'reminders'. Every notification you receive is an advertisement signalling a message to your brain.

When I was diagnosed with ADHD age 25, my life was in serious danger. I couldn't keep a job, maintain healthy relationships with family or friends, and kept spontaneously moving country whenever I had an issue, which led to some very dangerous situations. ADHD can be highly debilitating to live with, and waiting lists for NHS assessments in the UK are currently up to 7 years long, with private options costing thousands of pounds. I was diagnosed privately, and expected to pay £300 per month *for the rest of my life*, which is why I wrote *ADHD: an A to Z.*

An ADHD diagnosis can result in someone being legally considered to have a disability, which can be helpful to ensure people access the support they need and avoid discrimination, but with over half of the global population using social media, what happens if *everybody* becomes disabled? What happens if our brains are being deliberately rewired by technology acting completely within the law?

When I was growing up, I didn't know anyone who had any kind of mental health condition, but now almost entire classes are diagnosed. Parents tell me how their childrens' schools say there's nothing they can do about the fact they're all self-harming, and I hear on a near-daily basis about how educational institutions are failing students who desperately need support, because they're so overwhelmed.

ADHD symptoms can make you feel like you can't trust yourself, think through decisions, or communicate properly, as your mind is always racing ahead to the next thing. It's easy to lose track of who you are and what you want, because you're so easily distractable. 'Boring' things such as cooking, cleaning, administration and organisation can feel impossible, because our brains simply don't care. There are lots of brilliant things about having ADHD, but the symptoms of it shouldn't be imposed on us all by technology. Our ability to pay attention is a crucial part of being human and co-ordinating as a society, and if it's being so drastically damaged by technology, a wider conversation needs to happen about how we can all be supported, instead of facing 7 year waiting lists to access stimulant medication to help us cope.

Tips

- Treat any platforms profiting from your attention with caution, questioning everything you're shown, including posts, news and search results.
- Track your screen time across all your screens, not just your phones.
- Use apps such as 'Freedom', which enable you to block certain apps across devices.
- Turn off features that allow your activity to be tracked for the purposes of targeted advertisements.

- Charge phones outside of the bedroom at night, preferably all in the same place, at the same time – and buy an alarm clock!

- Have a 'phone box' that phones can be placed in, for example, next to the front door. You can also use a 'phone safe', which locks phones away for a specified length of time.

- Turn off notifications, including those on laptops (such as emails!), and for messages. Pick certain times of the day to check your messages rather than being accessible throughout the day.

- Use the grayscale mode on your phone to switch off the stimulating colours.

- Hide apps from your phone screen or delete them entirely – social media tends to be a lot less exciting on a desktop browser, without addictive features such as seamless scrolling.

- Block problematic websites on the browser on your phone.

- Get help from a professional if needed, such as a therapist or coach.

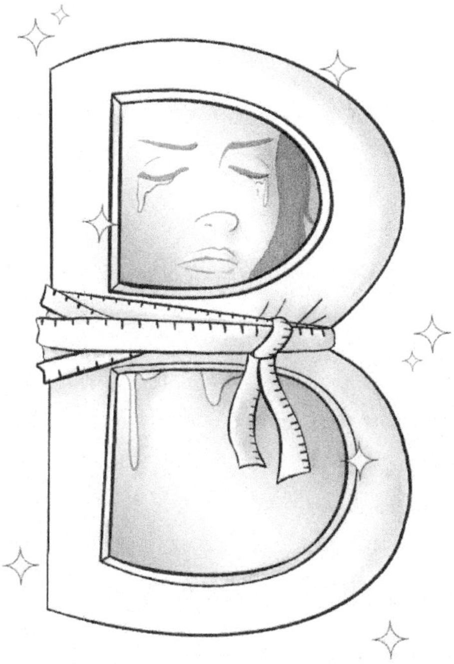

is for Beauty

B is for Beauty

Did you know?

- Facebook knows it makes body image issues worse for 1 in 3 teen girls.[4]

When they were teenagers, our grandparents probably saw as many 'beautiful' women in one year as we see in one hour on social media. Throughout my childhood, I was bullied for being ugly, until I turned 13, when my mum signed me up to a modelling agency. I really didn't want any more attention on my appearance, but I was booked on a photoshoot before being asked – it was just assumed that I'd want to be a model.

The job was a womenswear campaign, and the pictures were published in *Vogue*. This didn't magically make me feel beautiful, but it did make me feel safer against being bullied for being ugly, because I could point to a socially acceptable version of myself in a magazine, even if it looked nothing like me in real life.

In becoming a model, all that had changed was some random stranger's opinion of me. Being made over by experts and having my photograph taken by a professional photographer, with the final images edited and put into magazines, simply gave me a new standard of 'beauty' to compare myself to. I only saw this fake version of myself as acceptable, which made me hate the 'real' me.

---

[4] Damien Gayle, 'Facebook aware of Instagram's harmful effect on teenage girls, leak reveals', The Guardian, 14 September 2021. Accessed 10 March 2022: www.theguardian.com/technology/2021/sep/14/facebook-aware-instagram-harmful-effect-teenage-girls-leak-reveals

This is what we're all experiencing now: the ability to compare ourselves to a filtered version of ourselves that doesn't exist in reality. Social media apps can provide the same standard of makeover that I receive in several hours on a photoshoot in *seconds*. This can even happen without our consent or knowledge, with some social media apps featuring in built 'beauty enhancers'.

With a swipe of my finger, I can give myself a nose job, enlarged eyes, spotless skin, laminated eyebrows, a different hair colour, freckles, a new dress size, whitened teeth, thicker eyelashes, and more. Although no Photoshop skills are required for digital retouching apps such as Facetune, many of these features are built into social media platforms by the option to try out 'filters', which offer endless choices of pre-set versions of yourself.

Ten years ago, I used filters that gave me animal ears because they also smoothed out my skin, whereas today, it's popular to see ones with names such as 'VS Model'. This sets a dangerously impossible standard of beauty for us all to aspire to, because it doesn't exist. No matter how hard you try or how much money you have, all the cosmetic surgery in the world won't be able to remove the pores in your skin.

I've had messages from teenage girls telling me they can't bear to look in the mirror because they prefer the edited version of themselves. I understand this, having previously become so obsessed with editing the online version of myself to precise proportions, that I was convinced other people would be able to tell if I posted a photo of me that didn't match up to the edited version. Using filters became an addiction that I felt locked into, and I could no longer stand the real life version of me, feeling like I was living a lie.

Beauty standards

The definition of beauty is 'features or objects that are pleasurable to perceive', but to *whom?* Fashion magazines? Designers? I remember as a child, boys in my class rating the girls out of how attractive they were, and us girls being disgusted and curious at the same time. Their opinions mattered, because we weren't sure were else to find them - just like being a 'model' seems to give an objective stamp of beauty, regardless of anything else.

As in 'O is for Objectification', when the external version we present of ourselves to the world becomes so disconnected from our internal perception of who we 'really' are, our mental health begins to suffer. Social media gives us the illusion of controlling these measures in ways we've never been able to before, interpreting the instant feedback on the curated versions of ourselves as the personalized standards of 'beauty' imposed on us. It can feel like getting feedback on a school essay, with detailed instructions of how we could 'improve' ourselves next time, but the teacher will always find something wrong with us, no matter how hard we try.

The only reason that we equate models with beauty is because that's what we're told. Models aren't 'discovered', they're *manufactured.* Even if they're 'scouted' and invited to meet with a model agency, this doesn't mean anything – there's still a strong chance they'd be rejected, by these people who've invited them in! It's like someone approaching you in the street and inviting you for an interview to become a lawyer with a top city law firm – it wouldn't happen.

I was scouted when I was 18 in a shopping centre, and said I wasn't really interested, as I'd just started university. The scout persuaded me to meet with the top London agency, who after measuring me, told me to lose 3 inches off my hips to join them, even though I was already very thin! I said no and left in tears, but the scout called me and said she was worried about losing her job if I didn't do it as they hadn't accepted anyone that she'd scouted all year, so please could I try? Apparently, all I'd have to do was 'eat healthily for a few weeks', so I tried.

6 months of weekly measuring sessions, disordered eating, 'clothes shopping', expensive hair appointments and overall misery later, the

agency announced I was ready to start working, instead of just doing unpaid 'test shoots' at photographers' houses for my portfolio. Except, the photoshoots they'd booked me on for top magazines weren't paid, because 'high fashion, like magazines and catwalk, don't pay, and we're a high fashion agency.' When they asked me to lose 2 more centimeters off my hips to join their mainboard, I realised it would never end, and finally left, asking myself:

Why would anyone do a job where they have to change themselves completely, and not even be paid for it?

I hated how I looked with my dyed hair, bony body, and hungry eyes. After months of tweaking me like their own Barbie doll, this agency finally deemed me 'beautiful' enough to be privileged enough to work for free for some clients, but I'd never hated my appearance more. It's like having your self-esteem taken hostage by strangers, without even realising, or knowing what you're doing it for.

Today, social media operates just like this agency. It tells us how we should look, who we should be, and expects us to work for free. We're tricked into believing there's an end goal, and that it's helping us, but our self-esteem is being eroded with every 'beauty enhancer' tip we see.

Being an agency-signed model, just like being a 'blue-tick verified' influencer, is simply another rung on the ladder of validation. Just like anybody can set up a model agency from their bedroom, anybody could buy hundreds of thousands of fake followers on social media, as in 'I is for Influence'. This simply sets new standards to meet as in 'E is for Expectations' – whether that's consistently booking jobs or posting popular content. Each job or post can feel like it's your last one, because a 'million people would kill for your job' – just look at how many seasons of *Next Top Model* and *Love Island* there are!

This life is paved with insecurity, as in 'Z is for Zen', where you have to constantly worry about 'proving' yourself to both everybody you know in real life, and your imaginary audience online. If you want to become a model, or an influencer, ask yourself **why.** What's at the end of it?

The same goes for beauty standards. All I had to measure my self-worth on as a model when I was younger was how I looked, which is what many people using social media experience today. However, after writing 'the Model Manifesto', I've now got a permanent reminder that the rejection I experience as a model is often nothing to do with how 'beautiful' I am, but more likely to do with things such as rates and dates. The same goes for social media, such as dating apps and posts that don't 'do well' – this is nothing to do with how you look, and everything to do with the technology behind it, as in 'A is for Algorithms'

Our brains are constantly making up stories, and it's up to us whether to believe them or not, and whether to allow a social media platform to hijack what we believe to be beautiful. I've worked with some of the world's top supermodels, and I didn't think they were any more beautiful than the people I know in real life. To me, my friends and family are more beautiful than my colleagues, such as the creases in their face as they laugh, the glow radiating from their skin, and their eyes looking into mine.

This is beauty to me – not collar bones, foundation, or plastic. It's up to you to find that definition for yourself, but please don't let it be chosen for you.

Why are some platforms so bad for our body image?

Apps that focus on photos and videos (instead of words or sounds) are visual, so are focused on appearances by their very nature. Even if we don't post on these platforms, over a third of our brain's processing systems are dedicated to vision, and so what we see will have a significant impact on us.

Posting content allows a user to create a visual 'highlights reel' of their life, and features such as filters allow them to try out different features, from animal ears to new noses. They might feel more compelled to share this due to the novelty and wanting to share this experience with other people. However, just like being scouted by a model agency, this is where the insecurities start, because we're hoping for a reaction from the external world about how we look, as in 'V is for Validation'. This reaction, such as a certain number of likes or followers, can then be processed by the brain to be a direct equation of how attractive or popular we are.

The algorithms driving this are biased to get the maximum engagement from the user, with their own definition of beauty as 'what will get engagement', which can easily become our own. On social media, each post is already old news, and simply a new standard to keep up with – it will never be enough and can lead to unhealthy comparisons with others. Once you hit one goal, there's another one to reach. A target of 100 likes becomes 1000, which turns into 10,000, and so on.

People are nudged to post photos of themselves with tools like filters and algorithms that promote selfies, because we're always available. We live in a beauty-obsessed, capitalist world, and rather than waiting for luxury holidays or brunches to photograph, why not ourselves? As in 'O is for Objectification', when we start externalising our appearance to the world, we lose ownership and connection over it. We can start to measure our self-worth by how many likes a selfie gets, instead of how we genuinely feel about ourselves.

The issue with social media is that like capitalism, it will always keep us feeling badly about ourselves to keep us coming back. It not only promotes a largely fake world, such as my 13 year old self in womenswear campaigns, but it amplifies and targets this in extremely clever ways, 24 hours per day. Just like those women could never achieve my pre-pubescent body, we will never be able to achieve the filtered versions of ourselves we see on social media – they simply do not exist. If we all woke up happy with how we looked, entire billion-dollar industries would crash overnight. How would your life change?

Tips

- Look in the mirror and spot something you think is beautiful about yourself every day. If you struggle, just notice something you feel grateful to your appearance for each day.
- Make a beauty vision board of people you know in real life. What do you define as beautiful? How does this compare with what you see on social media?
- Try to remind yourself that filters are designed to make you feel bad about yourself, not good. When you're tempted to use them, ask yourself why, and consider speaking to someone about this.
- Spend time engaging with your own appearance in a way that feels good, such as by getting your nails or hair done, without posting it online.
- Try to notice if you make a negative comment about your appearance, and replace it with something you're grateful to that body part for instead, such as an experience it's allowed you to have.
- Try to notice your thoughts and comments about your own or other people's appearances, especially if you're around children. As above, you could set an example by consciously replacing it with something you're grateful to that body part for.
- Consider what you'd change about your own appearance. Why is this? How would life be different? Often there's a root cause behind what we'd like to change in life to become 'happier', so how could you address this root cause? For example, if you'd like more friends, could you join a new

social club? Get very specific on *why* you'd want to change how you look to understand what would make you feel better right now.

- Try to identify what makes you feel negatively about your appearance. For example, is it comparing yourself to other people? How helpful is this for you? If you can, try to identify a way to intercept these behaviours.

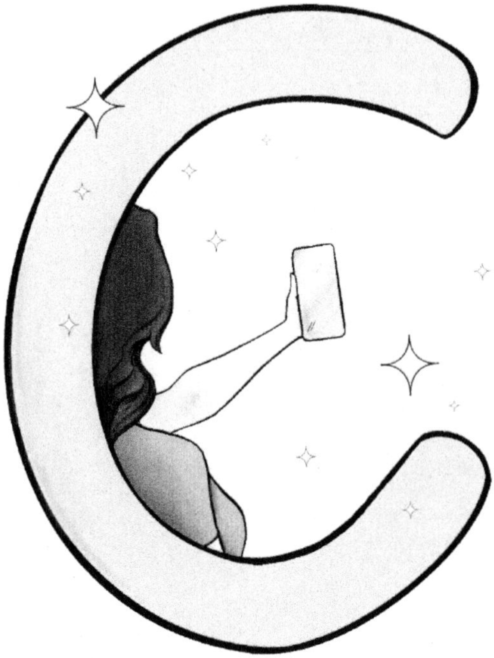

is for Content

C is for Content

Did you know?

- Advertisements by a medical company linking ADHD to obesity promoting negative body image were promoted on TikTok and Instagram, with no disclaimers.[5]

If social media is the cigarette that gives us cancer, content is the tobacco. Engaging with information online is how we stay feeling 'cool', though in many cases it can be just as pointless. The second we see a post, it's already old news. It's little wonder that nothing is ever enough, when the algorithms managing this content do it in a way that keeps us hooked, just like nicotine.

As we're all wired to be alert to threats to our safety, we're more likely to pay attention to negative rather than positive content, which is exploited by alogrithms seeking to keep us 'engaged'. They're not showing us content we *like* so much as content that will keep us returning to the platform, which is why there's so much negative and harmful content online. Viral videos of terrorism, hate speech and mass online trolling, to name just a few examples, show how dangerous the online world can be – essentially any information in the world is just a few clicks away.

Laws such as the UK's Online Safety Bill try to focus on content, but the content itself isn't the issue: the algorithms are. Ex-Facebook employee Frances Haugen explained how this works in the context of eating disorders, 'as young women begin to consume [this] content,

---

[5] Urian B, 'Ads Linking ADHD and Obesity Pulled from Instagram and TikTok | Cerebral Chief Medical Officer Says He Didn't Approve' | Tech Times, 27 January 2022. Accessed 17 March 2022.

they get more and more depressed. And it actually makes them use the app more. And so they end up in this feedback cycle where they hate their bodies more and more.'[6]

Content offers us both the problem and the solution. Just like Coca Cola a 'Diet' option, social media companies offer an endless vortex of information to keep us using. Whilst we've got the choice of what to consume, if our basic human vulnerabilities are being manipulated by powers we don't understand such as algoirthms, this choice is nothing more than an illusion. Presumably this is why drugs such as heroin are illegal but others are not: because they're inherently more addictive than human willpower.

Even the creation of this content, rather than viewing it, can result in harmful behaviours. For example, the most exciting part of my day on huge-scale production photoshoots used to be taking a selfie in the bathroom, after my hair and make up had been done by professionals. I'd feel the high of posting it online, but within minutes, I was anxious, constantly refreshing the page to check how much engagement it had received. Within an hour, I was low again, refreshing my emails in the hope of receiving another booking so that I could post another selfie 'proving' that I was working, and therefore 'beautiful', as in 'B is for Beauty'.

Every second we're spending thinking about, creating, viewing, or engaging with content for social media, we're subconsciously attaching a set of expectations to this. We're externalising our creativity and consuming others' through the medium of platforms biased to make us feel certain ways, distorting our sense of self-worth and validation.

---

[6] Kari Paul and Dan Milmo, 'Facebook putting profit before public good, says whistleblower Frances Haugen', *Guardian*, 4 October 2021, accessed 20 February 2022. www.theguardian.com/technology/2021/oct/03/former-facebook-employee-frances-haugen-identifies-herself-as-whistleblower

Living for content

When I graduated from university, I didn't know what to 'do' with my life. Without realising, I just decided to do what looked coolest on Instagram, moving to Australia, and seeking out the most popular spots for photos, doing photoshoots on the beach, and looking like I was living the dream. In reality, the better my life looked, the more I became depressed.

Living through my own Instagram lens didn't make me happy, but I couldn't stop. I was consumed with non-stop thoughts about what to post each day, obsessing over my numbers of followers and likes, constantly comparing myself to others. Whenever I wasn't on my phone, I felt like I was in almost physical pain. I had no idea who I was or what to do with myself when I wasn't posing for my imaginary audience, or trying to figure out how to become someone else – reality didn't seem to be an option for me anymore.

I started seeking out posts labelled with #triggerwarning, as an attempt to make myself feel better by comparing my depression to others. Instead, viewing this content made me become suicidal, as the deeper I fell into the vortex, the more it sought me out in return. I lost days of my life in bed endlessly scrolling through graphic content about how to kill myself, stuck in a vicious cycle of ruminating. It only stopped when I deleted my entire account.

Whilst it's great that mental health is more widely spoken about today, if this is being exploited in a way to profit from and exaggerate the insecurities and fears of other people, it can be very problematic. If social media companies were unable to profit from targeted advertising, then they may be able to provide much better quality information, such as how to get help (which would probably involve less time on social media!), but unfortunately, the aim is to keep you scrolling for as long as possible.

It's easy for anybody to fall into the same trap that I did, living for content and how things look, rather than how they actually are in reality. Just go to any concert or museum and see how many people experience these things through their phones, rather than being present. This is really sad, because it stops us from being able to genuinely enjoy life, and all the experiences it comes with. The best experiences in life, such as being around people we love, are impossible to summarise up in a photo or caption, and it's only by having them, that we grow as people.

Medium, not the message

Social media puts a huge amount of expectations and pressures put on us all that life should feel as good as it looks online, leaving us constantly disappointed. With so much access to information, we may believe that we should be able to reach the same standards as what we see online, even though these don't exist in reality. For example, if we actively see the 'morning routine' of celebrities, we might excitedly purchase the same products without a second thought.

20 years ago, we might have seen these standards whilst driving past a billboard, or when reading a magazine, but today, this content seeks us out 24 hours a day, deliberately targeting us with thousands of invisible adverts personalized to our unique vulnerabilities. Photo editing has been around for as long as digital cameras. However, our brain registers a gigantic billboard, or glossy magazine advert, very differently to a social media post. Whilst we might consciously be able to identify that a size 0 catwalk model is unrealistically thin, the same sized model appearing in a 'natural' Instagram post might be very different.

Social media can make companies act like individuals, and individuals act like companies by 'branding' themselves, as in 'O is for Objectification'. This means that it can be extremely hard to tell the difference between adverts that have been paid for by companies, although it's safe to assume that everything we see is being deliberately *shown* to us, whether that's by an algorithm or a deliberately curated highlights feed.

As in 'M is for Money', every second you spend online, social media platforms can collect your data to build a profile on you, which advertisers can then use to target you based on your 'interests'. Understanding what you're interested in means understanding your vulnerabilities. Whilst targeted advertising has existed for years in various forms, it can be extremely dangerous when combined with algorithms, as it can seek us out relentlessly in invisible ways, poking and prodding us until we give in and engage with the content.

We're also exposed to a lot more information about the people we know in real life online, who we might be more likely to compare ourselves to. If we're constantly seeing people we know using filters that remove pores from their skin or getting lots of followers, we might start thinking we should be doing the same. It's easy to forget that the content we see on social media has been curated to get a specific reaction, and may not be real at all. From watering down complex topics into a few words for infographics, or 'clickbait' articles, quantity of information definitely doesn't equate to quality.

The online world amplifies the same core principles of content that've always existed, but in a subtle yet all consuming way, leaving us blaming ourselves. It can be helpful to think of content as sugar: something that can be enjoyed in moderation, but to be mindful of. We're processing so much information every time we open up our screens that it's important to be in control of it – not the other way around.

Tips

- How present are you when having certain experiences such as going on holiday? What would it be like to have an exciting experience without posting it online?

- Why do you post content online? What are your motivations? Can you identify an overall purpose, and ask yourself what your motivation is for every post that you share?
- How do you engage with online content?
- Can you deliberately try out a new experience without sharing it online?
- Consider what type of content you engage with the most on social media. How does it make you feel? Is there any way that you can engage with it in a way that feels more balanced, such as not using filters?
- If you use social media for business purposes, can you make lots of content in advance and schedule it out using a planner, such as Canva or Later?

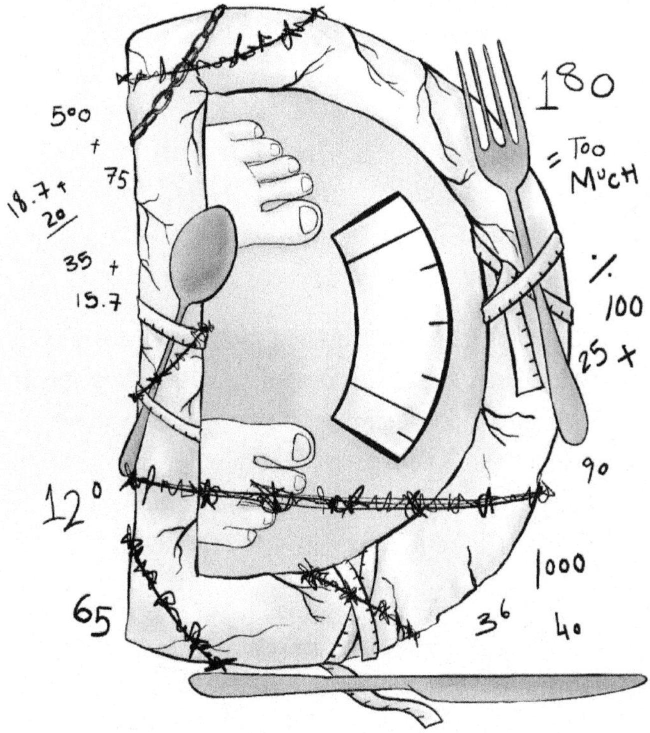

is for Disordered Eating

D is for Disordered Eating

- Facebook bought Instagram in 2012. During 2011/12, there were **2290** admissions to hospital for eating disorders, rising by 16% from the previous year.[7] In 2016/17, there were **13,885** admissions. In 2019/20, there were 20,647. In 2020/21, there were **23,302** hospital admissions in England for eating disorders.[8] **This is a rise of over 21,000 people in 10 years.** At the same time, obesity rates in the UK have almost **quadrupled** in the last 25 years, with 64.2% of the population being overweight.[9]

As social media enables and encourages us to compare ourselves to others, and unrealistic versions of ourselves, as in 'B is for Beauty', this can result in misguided attempts to control our inner or outer worlds in ways such as disordered eating. For as long as I can remember, there's been a silent yet obvious booming pressure in society to be thin, with the message imprinted into my brain that my weight was my worth.

This pressure can cause significant anxiety for us in a world where we're being constantly targeted with junk food advertisements and have more sedentary lifestyles than ever before, only made worse by the pandemic. For example, obesity levels amongst primary school children showed the highest annual increase of 4.5 points between

---

[7] BBC, 'Hospital admissions for eating disorders up by 16%' - BBC News, 11 October 2012. Accessed 17 March 2022.

[8] ITV, ''Hidden epidemic of eating disorders' sees dramatic rise in number, of children admitted to hospital' | ITV News, 4 January 2022. Accessed 17 March 2022.

[9] Obesity Statistics - House of Commons Library (parliament.uk), 16 March 2022. Accessed 18 March 2022.

2019-20 and 2020-21 since the National Child Measurement Programme began in 2006.[10]

For me, as I saw other girls in my class be bullied for being 'fat', especially by boys, I became obsessed with trying to keep my bony body as thin as possible, to avoid giving kids more excuses to bully me for how I looked. This only intensified when I became a model at age 13 and saw other teenage models being called fat and disgusting by model agents. However, sugar, like algorithms, can be stronger than our human willpower, and I often binge ate to make myself feel better – ironically putting on weight.

Even back then, the internet made things much worse. One day, when using the family computer, I somehow came across a 'thinspiration' website, promoting eating disorders. I knew instinctively that it was wrong and deleted the browser history. However, seeking this website out quickly became an addiction, as it provided me with step-by-step instructions on how to make myself sick, hide food, withstand hunger pangs, and stay motivated.

Every waking second was consumed with thinking about food, how to avoid it, and how to be thinner. These websites were behind my severe eating disorders, despite being very difficult to access due to my mum usually being in the room of the computer. They even had a fake page that could quickly be pulled up if somebody walked into the room!

Now compare this to today. I'd most likely have access to my own screen, especially in light of school classes happening online during the pandemic. If I came across these eating disorder websites, I'd not only be able to log in all the time, but I'd also be sought out by advertisements. I could be part of an interactive 'anti-recovery' community, sharing best practice with people I'd think were my

---

[10] Significant increase in obesity rates among primary-aged children, latest statistics show - NHS Digital, 16 November 2021. Accessed 18 March 2022.

friends, having my own accountability buddy to keep each other on track with our disordered eating.

I could hide my eating disorder much more easily behind normalised practices, such as following accounts on social media of people who are excessively thin, and put images of them as my phone background, or on my wall. I could try out filters that hollowed out my cheekbones and edit my photos to see how I'd look if I were size 0, literally being able to see my own 'goals', as this virtual version of me.

As in 'H is for Health', I could count how many calories were in every single item of food or drink I consumed, count the steps I'd taken each day, and build this up in my bedroom by doing exercise classes from the internet. Instead of just comparing my daily weight on scales, I could take daily photos of myself to compare myself to in minute detail. I could have easily framed this as being 'healthy'.

If I'd grown up ten years later, I probably would have died from an eating disorder by now.

Social media locks people into these illnesses, stamping them with an identity and perceived 'obligation', such as when vegan influencer Bonny Rebecca posted a video explaining her decision to eat meat again because of her severe health problems, receiving thousands upon thousands of comments of hate. The attention we get online can shape how we behave offline, which is especially dangerous when it's being distorted by algorithms promoting unrealistic and harmful content. Disordered eating far surpasses what we eat and becomes who we *are* – it becomes an identity.

For example, I know of a teenager whose selfies were shared thousands of times as 'thinspiration', which worsened her severe anorexia and cemented her with 'influencer' status. When she ended up in hospital and started to recover, she started receiving hate mail from other children who held her up as their inspiration for their own illnesses, calling her fat. This might seem incomprehensible, but when people are locked into all-consuming eating disorders, they lose the ability to be rational. Having had my own anti-recovery group in the form of a model agency determined to try and keep me as thin as possible, I've experienced first-hand how people can justify these bizarre behaviours towards others.

The illusion of control

As a model, I've never been weighed, but I have been expected to be able to make different parts of my body magically reproportion themselves, despite things like bone and organs being in the way. Despite this being impossible, the model agency tried to present the illusion of control by sliding a measuring tap around my hips every week. No matter how much I starved myself, I could not make the position of my bones change, and I'd usually binge on a box of chocolates on the way home out of shame and guilt.

This illusion of control underpins eating disorders, because it makes us think we might be able to reach this impossible goal, if only we try hard enough. Even though we might rationally know it's unrealistic to expect to look like people whose entire jobs are dedicated to looking a certain way, or who have digitally manipulated their photos, this doesn't stop us feeling bad about ourselves. People whose lives and identities are splintered on the internet may also have completely different perceptions of what is 'realistic', as in 'C is for Content'.

If we can create pictures of ourselves looking completely different to how we appear in real life, we might work towards this version of ourselves, especially if they receive a lot of attention online. I was *obsessed* with editing my photos to be perfectly proportioned, making my chest bigger and waist smaller, which made me hate my body in real life. My body image became so distorted that I believed people would think I was lying on social media if they met me in real life, even though the changes I was making were probably hardly noticeable to other people.

In this way, someone can easily develop **Body Dysmorphic Disorder**, where they believe there is something wrong with their appearance and obsessively try to 'fix' themselves. This may easily be amplified by existing harmful practices in the fashion industry, for example, such as models of maternity clothing wearing fake 'bumps' instead of being pregnant. It's easy to see how a pregnant woman could become obsessed with believing there was something 'wrong' with them because the images of apparently pregnant models they're seeing are so different, such as not having any swollen ankles!

The average dress size in the UK is 16, but plus size modelling starts at a size 12. My friends who were 'curve' models were under a lot of pressure to put *on* weight, and sometimes to had to take their own padding to photoshoots. Other 'diverse' categories such as 'petite', and 'tall' (both of which my pictures have appeared under on the same websites!) can simply be like producing different editions of Barbie dolls, using the same basic format. The reality is that the customer is still being misled and will never look like the Barbie personalized to them, no matter how much they might feel like they should identify with them.

Puberty also has a significant role to play. For example, as girls know their bodies will change as they go through their teenage years, they may try to hold it off – I certainly did. As in 'X is for X-rated', this might be understandable considering how sexualised their adult bodies can become, in a way that is completely outside of their control. This seems to be mirrored in the fashion industry, as 56% of models start working as children, and face pressure to keep their bodies in this child-like state, which is held up to society by capitalism as 'aspirational'.

Labels

Disordered eating can come in a variety of forms:

- **Anorexia Nervosa** relates to an obsessive desire to lose weight by refusing to eat.

- **Bulimia** relates to someone making themselves sick, typically related with binge eating.
- **Binge Eating Disorder** relates to someone eating a large quantity of food over a short period of time until being uncomfortably full.
- **Other Specified Feeding and Eating Disorders** is a catch-all classification covering a wide variety of behaviours, such as an excessive need to 'burn off' calories consumed.
- **Avoidant Restrictive Food Intake** relates to when a person restricts their eating, but not because of their body shape or fears of fatness, but they don't consume enough calories.
- **Pica** is an eating disorder involving eating items that aren't typically considered food and don't have nutritional value, such as eating paper, hair and ice.
- **Rumination Disorder** involves the regular regurgitation of food that occurs for at least one month, such as food being re-chewed or spat out.
- **Unspecified Feeding or Eating Disorder** relates to symptoms that cause significant distress but do not meet the full criteria for any of the 'disorders' listed above, usually because there's not enough information available.

The one thing I believe, with my lack of medical expertise, but significant personal experience of the above, is that **these are all largely the same thing: an emotional desire to control our bodies.** We might believe that by controlling our bodies, we can control our lives.

As a teenager, I made myself sick, spat out my food, eaten paper, taken diet pills, binged on chocolate, starved myself, tensed my stomach all the time to try and get 'abs', hid food in napkins, and went on diets. This didn't always show up as one of the above – I simply had disordered eating and needed help.

Today, social media can distort disordered eating even more. Influencers might be selling laxatives in the form of 'detox teas', or models might share 5 second videos of what they eat in a day. There's a never-ending stream of available workout videos and nutritional information, presented as being 'healthy' infographics. Restrictive diets might be framed as moral obligations, such as only living on fruit and vegetables. Impossibly proportioned people might be celebrated for how beautiful they are, despite refusing to admit to any surgery or editing of their photos, as in 'S is for Surgery'. The structure of people's faces might be automatically changed by filters on social media, and we might see adverts for weight-loss tablets, but all of this is completely normalised. Who are we going to complain to?

Ultimately, this can lead us to believe that we should be able to control their bodies in the same way as they can on the internet, but we just can't. The metrics of numbers such as followers and likes on social media can easily morph into the metrics of measurements, calories, and kilograms. This is a horrible, debilitating way to live – and it's never somebody's fault.

How to help

As a someone who's experienced disordered eating, I know how it can feel like you're being controlled by invisible powers, which you might not understand yourself, let alone be able to explain to other people. In a world that feels uncontrollable, believing that you can control at least what goes into your body might feel like a tiny form of emotional release, however how horrible it might be to experience. It can feel as though the only connection you have with your body, and become your entire identity.

Eating disorders are **emotional disorders** and need to be treated as such. We have to be able to recognise the problem in order to do something about it. I understand first-hand how external attempts from others to try and control your eating disorder can feel almost life-threatening, and how it almost makes it even more aspirational, because it signifies things must be working if other people are noticing. When someone's trying to take away that tiny morsel of control, it's easy to lose all rationality and try to hold onto it as hard as you can.

If you're experiencing this, or know someone who is, please try to remember that disordered eating is an illness, one which takes up a huge amount of brain power and energy. If you're trying to help someone, try to remember that although it might be very difficult, any anger or frustration you show towards them may only make it worse – they can't help it. There may be no clear identifiable reason behind this behaviour, and no apparent problem to solve – it's an illness, not a choice.

This makes tackling it very challenging, because it's so invisible. For example, asking someone if they've made themselves sick when they've disappeared at a dinner table, may make them feel embarrassed and angry (and they're unlikely to admit to this anyway). Sitting outside their bathroom door after dinner trying to catch them out may be pointless if you're not sure what to do if this happened. Checking up on a person might encourage them to devise even cleverer ways of hiding their behaviours. Forcing someone to sit at a table until they've eaten their dinner may just result in them becoming even more determined to burn the calories off.

People with disordered eating desperately need kindness, compassion, and understanding. They're in emotional pain, and need someone to speak to about it. By dealing with the underlying issues, such as a fear of being bullied if they put on weight, for example, the root causes can be solved. If you're going through this, try to find someone who you can speak to without judgement, and remember that there's always support available: you are not alone, and there's honestly more to life than this. The people who care about you are there for you – you don't need to worry about worrying them. Shame and silence are what binds us into pain – what you're going through is **not your fault.**

From my personal experience, I'd recommend focusing on these underlying emotional issues rather than calories, diet or weight, as this can just provide a different means of control, addressing the symptoms instead of the causes. Just like followers and likes, we can measure our self-worth by these numbers, despite them often being just as meaningless. Muscle weighs more than fat, and weight impacted by all sorts of things, including water intake and menstruation. When a friend of mine was suffering with her body image, we smashed her scales in the street with a hammer, liberating her from this daily habit. I really recommend you do thisor if you don't have any scales, find an equivalently liberating activity, such as ripping up fashion magazines and creating a paper-mache artwork!

There is hope. We might be living in a world of social media where there's an unbelievable level of scrutiny on our appearance, but we are first and foremost in the real world, where our worth is determined by simply existing. If you are a parent reading this book to try and help your children, please know how fortunate they are to have you caring about them.

<u>Tips</u>

- Smash your scales, delete your calorie counting and food delivery apps, and ditch your diets!
- Try to notice if you make comments about your own or other peoples' appearances. Where have these comments come from? Would you say them to a friend?
- Ask yourself what these comments mean, especially words like 'fat'. Question your thoughts to understand what you really mean by this: what are you really worried about?

- Try to speak to someone who won't judge you, and who you feel safe saying anything to. This could be a friend, family member, or therapist, for example. It can be really helpful to just speak and be listened to, to have your experiences validated.

- Try to find one thing you like about yourself every day. If this feels too difficult, try to identify one thing that you're grateful to your body for every day, such as keeping you alive.

- If people make comments about your appearance that feel triggering, explain how this makes you feel, and ask that the person stops making these types of comments.

- If you're part of any 'thinspiration' clubs on social media, I really cannot advise leaving them strongly enough. These people are unwell, and who want to keep you unwell, wasting your life obsessing about eating inside of living it. Don't let yourself be manipulated.

- Try out new activities where you use your bodies in different ways, such as going to a dance class, or joining a sports team.

- Remind yourself that feeling the way you're feeling is not your fault, and you have nothing to feel guilty for, just like a person with cancer.

- Try out cooking meals for yourself. If it seems too long winded, get a slow-cooker and throw some cans of food together – it's very easy! Try finding food you want to make, and enjoy the process of engaging with it in a present way, such as by noticing the smells and sensations in your body.

- If you don't like a certain food, try to think of how you could compromise on this, or try something you haven't had before.

- Avoid any measurements of your health, as in 'H is for Health', such as smart watches or apps that can track habits or calories

- Try yoga. A teacher I know called Emily Harding has online classes ('the Joyful Wild') appearing to focus on 'fitness', which she cleverly intertwines with body positivity. I used to think yoga was pointless, but slowing down and connecting with my body was a fundamental part of accepting myself. Ironically, the only thing we *can* control is our breathing, and how we react to things, which is what yoga is all about.

- If you're talking to someone with an eating disorder, I'd recommend asking as many questions as you can to understand what they're going through, and trying as hard as you can not to react or tell them what to do. I've learned the secret of coaching is asking questions that start with 'what', 'how', 'where', and 'when' – not why. These questions help a person get to that why by themselves, and 99% of advice given isn't taken.

- Seek professional medical help, including from a therapist.

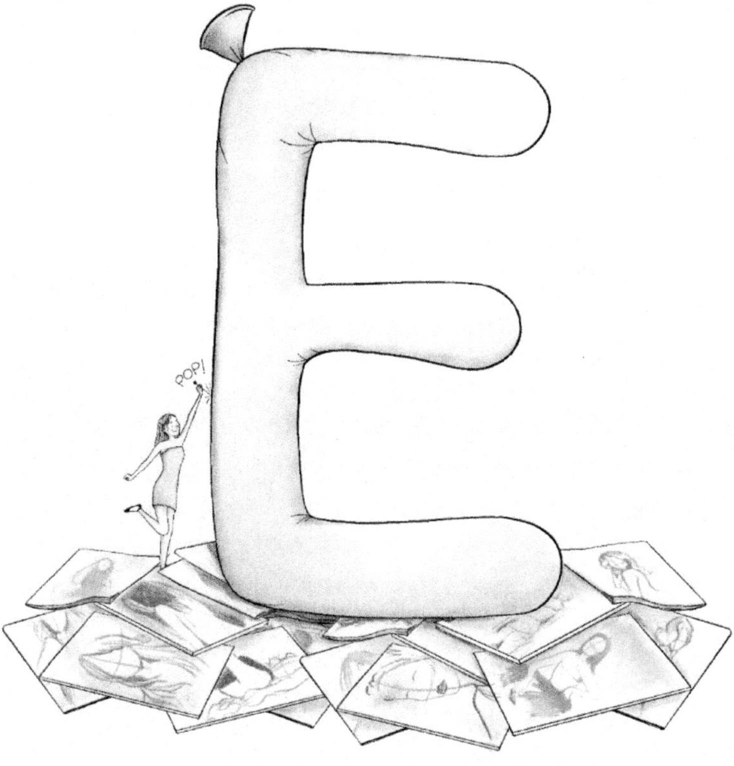

is for Expectations

E is for Expectations

Did you know?

- The suicide rate for women and girls between ages 10-24 increased by 94% since 2012, when Instagram became popular on a mass scale.[11]

For as long as I can remember, there's been two 'versions' of me: the real me and the model. We all have the experience of who we 'really' are and who we project externally to the world, but the wider this gap becomes, the more difficulty we can have with accepting our reality.

As a teenager, I'd compared myself to edited versions of myself in magazines, who I wouldn't have even recognised as me, if I hadn't been on the shoot. Throughout my modelling career, people have told me how I 'should' look and how I should edit myself in real life to match up to the ideal version of me they'd created in their heads. As in 'O is for Objectification', this made me disassociate from my body, losing any sense of ownership over it, and becoming depressed. I was burdened with the constant pressure of feeling like it should be different, but being unable to meet other peoples' expectations, no matter how hard I tried.

Social media gives us all this experience – of being presented with a 'better' version of ourselves and our lives, a perfected highlights reel that shows only the good times. When we set these unrealistic

---

[11] May Bulman, 'Suicides among teenage girls and young women have almost doubled in seven years, figures show', The Independent, 1 September 2020. Accessed 10 March 2022: www.independent.co.uk/news/uk/home-news/suicides-teenage-girls-young-women-rise-figures-a9698296.html

expectations on our reality, we're setting ourselves up for failure, because real life simply isn't as rosy as it looks on social media.

This can be especially confronting for young people who have grown up with the expectations that they should be able to match their 'real' selves with their 'social media' selves. They might even be able to track their entire lives through social media, right down to the day they were born, seeing a highlights reel of what appear to be their best moments throughout their life. The difference from looking at a photo album to Facebook is that they can measure their entire existence in external validation from other people.

Social media tells us we can do anything, be anyone, and achieve anything we put our mind to. It gives us a world of possibilities, from changing the shape of our body, to seeing what top celebrities eat in a day, or becoming a viral internet sensation overnight. It presents us with a literally never-ending reel of people to compare ourselves to, celebrating certain types of external achievements, and painting a picture of how life 'should' be, as in 'P is for Perfection'.

It can also be unforgiving, setting expectations that people could be 'cancelled' for making mistakes, as in 'R is for Resilience', and give the impression of a terrifying world, as algorithms show us content feeding our bias for negativity. Despite the world being objectively safer than ever before, social media can convince us that things have never been worse.

It's natural to feel overwhelmed at these expectations. When our 'external' self is so far from our 'internal' self, it means we must work harder to keep up with what we're presenting out to the world. For many of us today, these boundaries are blurred completely.

Filters

When Instagram brought out filters, I remember seeing them like virtual fancy dress, popping on bunny ears or turning myself into an alien. There was one which gave me dog ears and a lapping tongue, which airbrushed my face at the same time. I thought it made me look funny and cool, with the added highlight of being 'prettier'. It gave me a 'reason' to post, somehow feeling less arrogant than posting a normal selfie.

As in 'B is for Beauty', today, these 'fancy dress' filters have been largely replaced solely by 'beauty enhancing' features, that turn us into avatar versions of ourselves. The danger of this is that adults may see apps focusing on filters, such as Snapchat, as silly 'fun', but the digital versions that children are creating for themselves become expectations on who they 'should' be. Features such as 'disappearing photos' can also hide much more sinister uses of these apps, such as the expectation to send naked photographs, as in 'X is for X-rated'.

10 years ago, it felt shameful to edit my photos. I'd spend hours on an app called 'Airbrush', distorting my appearance, changing the shape of my features, editing myself to look how I thought I 'should' look. Today, it's completely different. Even professional apps such as Zoom come with 'beauty enhancing' options, my phone constantly suggests edits of my photos to me, and the 'plastic surgery look' is in high demand in the modelling world.

These filters make perfect business sense, because they might temporarily boost how a person feels about their appearance on the app, especially if they're activated without them even knowing. It's only when they log off and look in the mirror, that they feel might worse about themselves. It would be like going to a shop and fitting into clothes that are a size smaller to what you usually wear, despite there being zero standardisation between clothing sizes across brands!

We're all being offered a 'better' version of ourselves by technology, and don't think anything of it. As in 'S is for Surgery', one woman I know was offered a free beauty consultation, where photographs of her face were taken and blown up on a screen, with red lines drawn on to highlight her 'problem areas'. She left much poorer, with her self-esteem irrevocably damaged by having a stranger point out 'flaws' to her, some of which she'd never even thought about before stepping into that room.

Now imagine that happening multiple times a day. How would you feel if in real life, someone approached you and suggested you had a cosmetic surgery procedure to look better? How about if they asked you to lose weight? This is what happened to me at age 18 by a model scout who'd approached me in a shopping centre. Receiving backhanded criticism from others about our appearance, whether this is a person or technology, can have a lasting impact on your self-esteem and the expectations of how you believe you 'should' look.

Expectation Dysmorphia

If you're editing your social media content, it can be very difficult to stop, especially if you're getting positive feedback from the internet. The feedback we receive through this 'external' version of ourselves might feel much more exciting than our reality, as in 'V is for Validation'. When I was addicted to editing my content, I felt extremely anxious about people seeing me without this editing, or eventually, even in real life. It felt like everybody would be able to tell I was a fraud, even though the differences were hardly noticeable. These self-set expectations grew into obsessions and phobias of the real world, making me overthink things much more than anybody else would. It literally filtered my thoughts.

In 2020, unfiltered photographs of Khloe Kardashian in a bikini were accidentally posted, and quickly deleted, from her account. The photos were nothing shocking, but she looked much less like a fake Barbie doll than she did in other images. However, what *was* extraordinary was her reaction to this: an obscene amount of effort must have been made by her and her team in attempting to get these images removed from the internet, despite this being impossible and only drawing more attention to them.[12]

In comparison to walking past a photoshopped billboard on the street, it's like being photoshopped into it, and having it tattooed onto our eyeballs: having unrealistic expectations make feeling bad about ourselves inevitable. It can be both all-consuming and invisible to others, becoming all that we can think about. It's easy to trivialize this as being 'fun', or just being like using make up in real life, but that's the point – what happens if you can't leave the house at all because the only acceptable version of yourself is impossible to recreate?

This can also apply to our offline lives, as we might seek out new outfits to wear that haven't already featured on our social media, or feel unable to enjoy any experiences without thinking about how to post about it online, as in 'C is for Content'. When our filtered virtual reality is so extreme, living in the real world can pale in comparison, leaving us dependent on the highs of living vicariously through the seemingly more exciting lives of celebrities and other people we follow, rather than our own.

Just like Body Dysmorphic Disorder, feeling like this is not a choice – it's an illness. It can easily spiral into self-esteem issues and depression, and lead to wanting to live primarily through a screen, rather than in real life. For example, as a parent, I imagine it's very difficult to convince your child to do their maths homework instead of watching an endless stream of the inner lives of their favourite influencers – how do you argue with that? How do you convince them to go for a walk in the rain around the local park, when they could be virtually experiencing a luxury beach resort? Arguing for reality can be exhausting, but it's necessary, because these worlds aren't real.

---

[12] Paul Glynn, 'Khloe Kardashian tries to get unfiltered photo removed from social media', *BBC News,* 7 April 2021. Accessed 20 February 2022. www.bbc.co.uk/news/entertainment-arts-56660476

Fake expectations

The way content is consumed on social media has made fake expectations seem achievable. When model Kendall Jenner posted a 'behind the scenes' photograph from a shoot in 2021, I received messages from at least 10 different people telling me how much this photo had made them hate their bodies. The fact this seemed to be a 'casual' photo snapped quickly in a mirror was much more damaging than the final polished campaign images, because they seemed to imply this was achievable in 'real life'.

Even without images being digitally edited, professional models know how to position their bodies in ways to give an impression of looking a certain way. It is literally their job to look a certain way, and people like Kendall Jenner have most likely had years of personal training and nutritionists, at the very least. Although some adults might be able to make this distinction and rationally understand that this is an altered image in some way, younger people in particular might find it much harder – or they might not even care. They might feel inspired by believing this is possible to achieve, spurring them on more in their own pursuits to control their bodies, as in 'D is for Disordered Eating'.

Social media removes the distinction between adverts and reality, positioning our friends' selfies next to those of celebrities'. Whilst our brains would be better able to rationalise that what we see on a huge billboard has likely had a huge amount of investment into it and may not be achievable for us looking up at it, when it's shown via a square on our phone, this may make it feel achievable – especially if we're seemingly sold the 'how to' products or steps behind this. There's no proper regulation over this global wild west marketplace, which could, for example, result in people who've changed their body shape with surgery advertising shapewear underwear to their audience to look like them, without disclosing the surgery they may have had.

Misleading advertising laws exist for a reason – if we believe the fake expectations being advertised to us, we'll be trapped in a loop of self-hate, believing that it's our fault that our realities don't measure up. To believe that maybe our favourite influencers or apps don't have their best interests at heart can be monumentally overwhelming, especially when we may have built our entire identities around them. No matter how hard they try, we will never be able to meet these expectations, because they simply do not exist.

Tips

- Consider what you see on social media and how you feel about it.
- Do you use filters? Why? What effect does this have on you?
- Try to find a fun activity you might like to experience, and do this without taking your phone.
- Try a life drawing class – I found this one of the most helpful things I did for my own self-esteem. Classes such as 'Body Love Sketch Club' emphasise the importance of play, fun, and beauty in all of us.
- What expectations do you have of yourself? What do you think you 'should' be doing, feel, or look like? Are these expectations from you or from what you've seen on social media?
- What did you enjoy doing as a child? How could you do this activity again in some small way? So many of us lose this experience when we realise we can't be 'professionals', but can you just do it for fun, such as by taking a dance class?
- Notice when you say that you 'should' do something, and try to ask yourself whether you actually *want* to do it.
- Remember that you don't need to be 'successful' on social media to be successful – this book is an example!

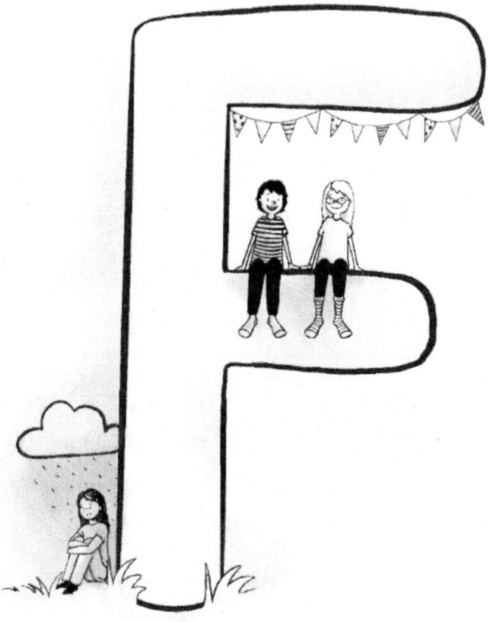

is for Friendships

F is for Friendships

Did you know?

- Around one fifth of the UK's population feel lonely, which can be as harmful to our health as smoking 15 cigarettes a day.[13]

As a child, if I wanted to see my friends outside of school, I had to call their house phone and ask to speak to them. I only knew about the meet ups I wasn't invited to by gossip in the classroom. If I didn't get a modelling job after going to a casting, I forgot about it soon enough.

As I got older, things changed. I started to post photos online I'd taken on a camera from meet ups with friends, as proof that I was 'popular'. I arranged meet ups with friends over text messages that costed 25p each. I started to see online Facebook events of parties, with long lists of invitees that didn't include my name. If I didn't get a job, I could watch it play out on Instagram as it happened, comparing myself to the model who had been booked instead.

It's easy to forget how much friendships matter when you're at school. How the opinions of this defined group of people can make or break you, because they feel like your only choice. It's also easy to forget how horrible kids can be to each other, for seemingly no reason at all, like me being relentlessly bullied for things outside of my control, such as my height.

However, social media provides the opportunity to be friends with the entire world. Whereas I was always told not to speak to strangers on the internet as a child, today, we're all having entire friendships

---

[13] Hannah Schulze, 'Loneliness: An Epidemic?', *Science In The News*, 16 April 2018. Accessed 20 February 2022.
www.sitn.hms.harvard.edu/flash/2018/loneliness-an-epidemic/

with people on the other side of the world. It's also never been easier to have relationships with people we know and never even see them in real life: our friendships are moving online.

Social media can also expand into all areas of our relationships with other people. When I was at school, I would have only known about a party that I wasn't invited to by maybe hearing other people ask if I was invited, or speak about it the Monday afterwards, but today, I can watch it play out in real time. I can keep track of my friends' online activity with each other, attempting to measure out whether I'm at risk of being liked 'less' than others, literally counting the number of likes and comments. It can easily become an obsession that we simply didn't think about as much in the days before social media.

This also goes for trolling and bullying, as in 'K is for Kindness', where we can be mercilessly targeted 24 hours a day, 7 days per week. Social media gives an entirely different context to relationships, making them potentially more transactional and fragile, but especially for younger people, who maybe haven't had the experiences of going through different life experiences with their peers.

Quality or quantity?

Although we've been able to connect with more people than ever before, this doesn't necessarily mean they're all our friends. Whilst it's obviously difficult to keep up with the lives of more than a handful of people on a regular basis, if we've got hundreds or thousands of online followers that we think are our friends, we may believe we *should* be able to maintain this many connections.

This can leave us feeling exhausted and burnt out. For example, influencer Molly Mae Hague said she has over 6 million followers on Instagram, but only 5 friends. Her millions of followers simply cannot give her the same level of understanding, compassion, support, and security as people who care about her in real life.

This can also be dangerous for people who trust what they see online, and can easily be manipulated into dangerous situations such as scams, as in 'M is for Money'. It can be hard to tell the difference between 'followers' and friends, and we may even prefer some people they speak to online, who might seem to understand the 'real' us better than those we know in real life.

When I had lots of Instagram followers, I believed these people were my friends. They weren't – they were my *audience.* They became the people I posted for, who I prioritized over my real-life relationships, because I was constantly chasing more hits of validation. The tools I was using to measure my own popularity were an illusion, because we can simply never feel properly fulfilled from online connection alone. The more followers we have, the lonelier and more disconnected from real relationships we can become. It can result in the belief that friendship can be measured by the amount people engage with each other on the internet, when in reality, friendship is so much more than this.

Communication

Having lots of connections presents the challenge of managing these relationships in a way that fits with the invisible rules of social media, from posting regularly, to commenting on each other's posts. As we have become accessible all day, every day, we might feel obliged to reply to hundreds of messages each day from different people, where conversations can lose their sense of meaning.

When I deleted my social media accounts, I realised I hadn't properly spoken to many of my friends in months, because we'd just fallen into a pattern of liking each other's posts instead. These relationships required more effort on both sides, needing us to have an actual conversation to stay in touch, rather than leaving a comment on a post.

Online communication can become quicker and quicker, turning into sped up voice notes monologuing about our days, without really listening to each other. Friendships like this can feel like the equivalent of junk food, because we're overwhelmed with excess, but never feel properly satisfied.

This can be dangerous for people who may appear to be extremely popular, but might be feeling lonely, which can be driven by expecting they *should* feel more connected than they do. They might be talking to many people at the same time, but still feel like they're not being heard, or their messages are being misunderstood, for example. Whereas it's become easier than ever to send a 10 minute voice note, just think how rare it is to receive a hand written postcard from someone we care about!

Rejection

Social media has put our friendships at risk of becoming transactional, where we meet up to 'create content', giving us 'proof' of being mutually liked. Whilst this might start out positively, when it becomes an obligation, or the entire purpose of our friendship, this can leave us with bad self-esteem, believing people only talk to us when there's something in it for them. This might not even be true, but we might struggle to relate to people in any other way. Having truly vulnerable, emotional, and connected conversations is becoming harder and harder in a world filled with so many distracted connections.

Social media also provides a breeding ground for measuring in precise detail how unliked we are, such as by using apps that send notifications when someone unfollows us. We might also feel rejected if someone we know in real life doesn't like our post(s), concocting an entire narrative in our head that doesn't exist, based around our worst insecurities. For example, I was always deleting posts that didn't get enough likes, and getting annoyed with my friends for not liking them. In reality, things are rarely as personal as they feel, but this is difficult to remember in a world where we're being deliberately made to think the opposite, as in 'A is for Algorithms'.

It allows us to conflate content with the person, and online likes with how much we're liked in real life. Having lots of notifications pop up when we post a picture can give the imagined effect of feeling loved and popular, but when we keep refreshing, and the notifications stop coming, we may feel low again, needing to post more to get the same high. People who don't live inside this bubble, who can't offer any highs or lows through this way, may become less exciting in comparison.

It can feel much easier to dig deeper into our holes of loneliness than expose ourselves to potential rejection by trying to meet up with someone in real life, and we might feel scared about what that might be like if we don't have a 'reason' for our friendship, like posting an experience online. Children may have grown up with this version of communication with others – they might not have ever felt the true benefit of having a 'real life' friend that genuinely cares about them. Friends allow us to have conversations and connections, which make us feel happy – they're vital to our wellbeing.

Fear of Missing Out / Loneliness

Being alone isn't necessarily the same as being lonely – just the expectation ourselves that we shouldn't be. For example, most of us wouldn't care if we didn't have plans on a Monday evening – but how about if this was a Friday or Saturday evening? The thought of other people out having fun with each other makes us feel like we should be too.

Social media has magnified the fear of missing out, whilst making us feel lonelier than ever, because we think we're alone in feeling this way. We can literally watch their friends hanging out with each other, hear about the Whatsapp groups we're not in, check who has watched our 'stories', and see the seemingly happy relationships of everyone else we know. This can make us feel as though everyone else is happy and connected, questioning what's wrong with us.

I felt incredibly lonely as a model living my top 'Instagram' life in Australia, because I couldn't stop focusing on my imaginary audience of friends rather than making real life connections. I was addicted to checking my likes, replying to text messages, and commenting on pictures, but these things didn't make me feel connected or popular – they just made me feel like I wasn't enough. Loneliness keeps us addicted to the cause, as we go on social media in attempt to connect with other people, leaving us even lonelier!

The secret to overcoming FOMO is that it's these social comparisons that make people feel lonely – if we don't know what's happening, we don't care. Social media gives us a window into anything we want to see – whether that's a celebrity's luxury holiday, what strangers are eating for breakfast, or the party we missed on the weekend. If we didn't see this, we wouldn't care, but instead we can subject themselves to the torture of watching other people's highlights reels of things that almost certainly aren't as much fun as they look.

We can invent all kinds of stories of the fun we've missed out on, and reasons we aren't having these experiences, beating ourselves up and fuelling our motivation to post more content as proof we're not missing out. However, the second that content is posted, its old news, and we're thinking about the next experience.

Social media can also allow people to compare their current life to their own previous personal highlights reel, such as wanting to go on an even more 'aesthetic' holiday next time than the one they've just been on. It can be easy to convince ourselves the antidote to loneliness is by growing our following, and making even more connections, but this will simply leave us more unhappy.

This is the reality of FOMO: nothing will ever make us feel like we're not missing out, because it's simply not possible to have all the experiences we see on social media, or be friends with all the people in the world. None of us will never have 'enough' friends, just different types of people to compare ourselves to. All we're really missing out on is the ability to enjoy the present moment as it is, and the people in our lives we've already got.

Tips

- Try to spend time with people in real life. It can be easy to de-prioritize friendships in a world obsessed with productivity, but try to ensure you have time to see the people who make you feel good about yourself every week.

- Identify 5 people in your life whose opinions you genuinely care about. Can you prioritize these people above everybody else?

- Consider how you feel about your followers online, and how these compare to your real-life relationships. How much energy do you give to both types of people?

- If you can, try to be conscious about how you're communicating with people. Do you feel heard in your relationships? How can you express your preferred method of communication to the people in your life?

- If you're feeling lonely, try to identify a real life activity where you can meet more people, such as attending a new club or group activity.

- Consider how good your friendships make you feel. Do you feel any pressures to like their posts? If you want to take a break from social media, can you explain this to your friends and think of different ways they can keep in touch with you?

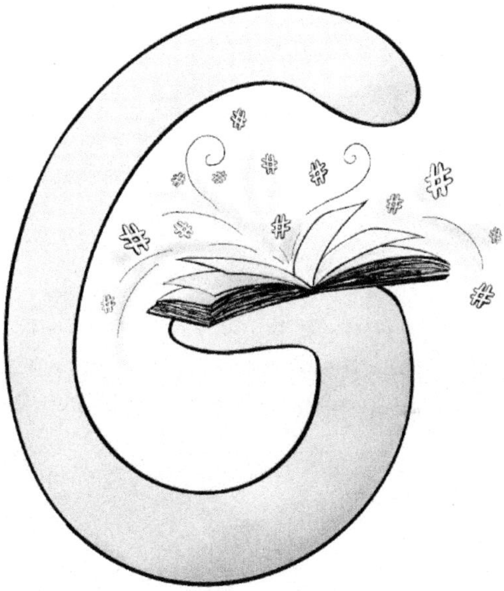

is for Glossary

G is for Glossary

Did you know?

- The cartoon character Winnie the Pooh was blocked in China because bloggers compared him to China's president.[14]

- **Ad:** an advertisement It's the business model of social media companies to profit from advertisements shown to people viewing their content, which could be obvious (e.g a clip showing before a YouTube video) or less obvious (e.g an influencer posting about a product they've been 'gifted' without making this clear).

- **Algorithm:** formulas developed for a computer to perform a certain function, such as promoting content that will keep users engaged for the longest amount of time.

- **Ana:** pro-anorexia websites refer to anorexia as 'Ana', usually referred to as 'pro-ana'.

- **Analytics (or 'Insights'):** data showing the performance of a person's social media page, such as how many views they've had, where their audience are based, and their 'engagement' rate when others are interacting with them online. Apps can allow users to track their analytics in precise detail, particularly if they have a 'business' account.

- **Anti-recovery:** communities of people typically supporting each other *against* recovering from mental illnesses, such as pro-eating disorder websites or groups on platforms such as

[14] Stephen McDonell, 'Why China censors banned Winnie the Pooh' - BBC News, 17 July 2017. Accessed 17 March 2022.

Facebook. They may coach each other on the most effective ways of staying unwell and hiding this from others, promote illnesses such as anorexia, compete by sharing metrics such as measurements, and could even have group sessions of activities such as self-harming. They could share information such as instructions on how a person can kill themselves and encourage each other to do it, adding people back into the groups who leave.[15] Obviously, these are extremely dangerous.

- **App:** a programme someone can download and use instead of going on a website through an internet browser. They tend to be less engaging on the browser!
- **Archive:** a feature allowing users to hide certain posts or messages in a different folder, such as on Whatsapp or Instagram.
- **BBL:** Brazilian Butt Lift surgery involving removing fat from a person and re-injecting it into their buttocks. This has become very popular on social media, with posts showing surgery transformations going viral.
- **Bio:** a short description of who someone is, as seen on social media profiles.
- **Bitmoji:** an avatar or emoji users can create to look like them, seen on apps like Snapchat.
- **Blog:** regular entries of content on a specific topic, description of events, or other resources such as graphics or video. Essentially, most social media websites.

---

[15] Monica Greep, 'Instagram algorithm pulls teenagers into suicide groups, says Facebook whistleblower Frances Haugen', Daily Mail Online, 7 February 2022, accessed 27 February 2022.

- **Business Account:** anybody can set up a business account on social media for free, which usually shows more detailed analytics.
- **Booed:** receiving negative comments on a post as disapproval.
- **Boomerang:** a short looping clip lasting for a few seconds.
- **Boomer:** broadly speaking, a 'baby boomer' can refer to any pre-millennial, which recently became very popular in relation to a phrase called 'OK Boomer', which essentially dismisses an older person's opinion. It's been referred to as a 'sophisticated, mass retaliation' against the impact of past generations.[16]
- **Bot:** a 'robot' or social media account that's been designed to post automatically for a specific purpose. Usually related to fake information, followers and engagement!
- **Brand rep:** a brand representative can be someone who receives a discount from brands for sharing about their company and is becoming more common to see on a micro-scale.
- **Cancel(led):** essentially this is to stop supporting a person, possibly calling for everyone else to 'cancel them' as well, making them irrelevant. This could be the digital version of 'no-platforming' someone, in preventing a person with certain views from contributing to a public debate or meeting, especially one which they'd been previously invited to attend.

---

[16] Joshua Bote, 'Why are Gen Z and millennials calling out boomers on TikTok? OK Boomer explained', Receive News, 4 November 2019, accessed 27 February 2022. www.receive.news/11/04/2019/why-are-gen-z-and-millennials-calling-out-boomers-on-tiktok-ok-boomer-explained/

- **Chat:** as well as referring to messages between people, there may be 'Group Chats', such as on Whatsapp, which children might not always be included in.
- **Clickbait:** marketing or advertising material using sensationalized headlines to attract clicks.
- **Conversion rate:** the percentage of people who completed an intended action (e.g clicking on a link).
- **Connections:** when users connect with each other online. This might be a Facebook 'Friend', or LinkedIn 'Connection', for example, categorized by 'degrees' of how many people users know in common. Typically these are made by one person sending a 'Request'.
- **Content**: information posted online - as in 'C is for Content'.
- **Comment:** a response that is often provided as an answer or reaction to a post on social media.
- **Community (or Groups):** features on platforms where people with similar interests can join a group and discuss related topics, such as Facebook.
- **Creator:** the creator of content. It's worth noting here that apps such as TikTok have set up 'Creator Funds' to pay users with a certain number of followers and posts for their content based on views (which could explain its sudden mass popularity!).
- **Cyberflashing:** the act of sending sexually explicit photos or videos to someone else without their permission or knowledge. This can happen by being sent a photo over Bluetooth, for example.
- **Deep Fake:** media in which a person in an existing photo or video is replaced with someone else's likeness, a practice

becoming increasingly common, especially in relation to pornography.

- **Direct Message (DM):** private conversations occurring on social media accounts such as Twitter and Instagram. People don't necessarily have to be following each other, and a popular slang term is 'slide into my DMs'.
- **Discover:** a section of a social media platform dedicated to showing new content they might like.
- **Disappearing messages:** time sensitive content which typically disappears after a certain period, such as on Snapchat or Whatsapp.
- **Engagement:** the interaction between a person and a piece of online content, such as 'liking', sharing, commenting on, or viewing it.
- **Engagement pods:** groups of people who band together to help increase engagement on each other's content, such as all commenting on each other's posts.
- **Emoji:** small cartoonish images that can be sent to express emotions.
- **Fans:** people who like a certain page, such as on Facebook.
- **Fake news:** misleading information that is presented as news.
- **Facetune:** an app allowing a person to very easily edit their appearance, including changing the dimensions of their features.
- **Filter:** the ability for a person to edit their appearance by using pre-set 'filters' that can distort how they look, for example, by giving them animal ears or poreless skin. Social media platforms such as TikTok and Instagram have thousands of potential filters to choose from, which can be

created by users themselves (and so may be hard to moderate!).

- **Finsta:** short for 'fake insta', this describes a hidden Instagram account. It's good to note that people can have as many as they want!
- **Follower:** a person who subscribes to another's account to receive their updates. They could also be 'fans' if they like a certain page, such as on Facebook.
- **For You Page (FYP):** a hashtag TikTok users place in their videos to prioritize their content on other users' 'Your Page' feed. This feed shows people content uniquely tailored to what they're interested in, regardless of whether they're following the accounts or not.
- **Geotag:** a post sharing a location, such as where a photo was taken. It's obviously good to ensure children are aware of the dangers of sharing their location with strangers online, which can often be forgotten, even by adults!
- **GIF:** an acronym for Graphics Interchange Format – usually small animations lasting a couple of seconds long, that can often be used in private messages and easily created by users.
- **Ghosting:** the practice of ending all communication with a person without any apparent warning or justification, and ignoring them. This can often be related to modern dating.
- **Like**: features allowing people to demonstrate they approve of a post by 'liking' or favouriting it.
- **Handle:** the term used to describe someone's username, usually starting with an @ symbol.

- **Hashtag:** a tag used in posts starting with #, which categorizes information and makes it easily searchable to users.
- **Hinge:** a dating app (other popular ones at the time of writing include Tinder, Feeld, Raya, and Bumble), where people make profiles and 'swipe' left or right on a person to 'match' with those they like.
- **Instagram Live / IGTV:** where accounts can post longer-form videos of content, often broadcast live.
- **Impressions:** how many people have seen or interacted with a post.
- **Influencer:** a social media user with the potential to reach a relevant audience and create awareness about something. Usually referred to as 'mega' (celebrities), 'macro' (people with 100ks-millions of followers), 'micro' (typically between 1000-100k followers, maybe focusing on a niche subject), 'nano' (typically 0-1000 followers who have influence in their community), and 'virtual' – ones that are computer generated.
- **Instagram:** a popular photo-sharing app, featuring 'endless scrolling' of posts.
- **Last Seen:** a feature on apps such as Whatsapp which notifies the user when someone was last 'seen' online.
- **Like:** an action that can be made on social media showing that a person approves of a post.
- **Lighting:** some users may use professional lighting for their posts, such as by using a 'ring light', which can be attached to their phone.

- **LinkedIn:** a business-orientated social networking site, essentially showing online CV's. It seems to rapidly be becoming more popular with more personalized content, so it's good to note that this could be potentially vulnerable for people looking for jobs, as it's easy for others to appear very trustworthy and professional on this platform, and it's normal to 'connect' with people you don't know.

- **OnlyFans:** a social media platform allowing people to earn money from users who subscribe to their content (the 'fans'). This is commonly linked to posting and selling sexually explicit content. In May 2021, a BBC Investigation found under-18s had been bypassing age verification systems, with police saying children are being 'exploited' on the platform.[17]

- **Podcast:** audio files that are released by episodes, usually seen on platforms such as Spotify and Apple Podcasts. It's very easy to set up a podcast and they can be highly influential.

- **Pinterest:** a photo sharing network providing users with a platform for uploading, saving, and categorizing 'pins' through collections called 'boards'.

- **Marketplace:** platforms such as Facebook and Depop allow users to buy and sell items from each other.

- **Meme:** a post that is used to describe a thought, idea, or joke that's widely shared online, often with a photo or video and accompanying text.

- **Mention:** when a person is literally 'mentioned' or tagged by another user on a platform.

---

[17] Noel Titheradge and Rianna Croxford, 'The children selling explicit videos on OnlyFans', BBC News, 27 Mary 2021. Accessed 27 February 2022. www.bbc.co.uk/news/uk-572559

- **Metaverse:** a reference to virtual worlds where users can interact with each other and apps in a very immersive way. This is still very new, but the BBC has found that children are at serious risk, potentially being groomed, going to virtual strip clubs and acting out virtual sex.[18]

- **Misinformation:** misleading information presented as fact, which can commonly happen on social media given the lack of verification!

- **Mia:** this can be a reference to bulimia by eating disorder websites, also referred to as 'pro-mia'.

- **Notifications:** alerts about updates, often appearing in 'bubble' format and igniting the curiosity of a person to go on the app to view it in full.

- **Nude:** a sexually explicit photo or video of someone. Often heard in the phrase 'send nudes'.

- **News Feed:** literally, a feed full of news, showing all the latest updates since a user last logged in, and typically not in a purely chronological way. Also referred to as a 'Timeline'.

- **Reddit:** a social news site containing various specific topic-orientated communities of users who share content on forum messaging boards. Topics ('subreddits') can be very niche!

- **Selfie:** a photo that someone takes of themselves, usually by using the reverse camera on a smartphone, orby using a selfie stick (a pole that attaches to their camera).

- **#selfharm(mmm):** a hashtag where people share photos of their self-injury, possibly adding letters on the end to avoid posts being blocked.

---

[18] Angus Crawford and Tony Smith, 'Metaverse app allows kids into virtual strip clubs', BBC News, 23 February 2022. Accessed 27 February 2022. www.bbc.co.uk/news/technology-60415317

- **Share:** when one users shares or reposts another's content (also 'Retweeting).
- **Snapchat:** an app that allows users to share time-sensitive photos and videos known as 'snaps', which disappear after a certain period but are still stored on the Snapchat server. This is commonly associated with using filters and sending inappropriate content.
- **Snap Map:** a feature of Snapchat that allows users to see where their friends are, as well as hot spots where people are publicly posting stories.
- **Stan:** to be an obsessive fan of a particular celebrity.
- **Story:** a post / series of posts on a platform such as Facebook or Instagram that typically last for 24 hours. These can be public or shared only with certain people.
- **Spon:** sponsored content. If a user has been paid to post content, there are rules saying they should make this clear by hashtagging #ad or #spon in their post.
- **Spotify:** a music streaming service where users can listen to podcasts and songs, and share what they're listening to with other people / see what their friends are listening to.
- **Swipe up:** a feature allowing users with over 10,000 followers and a business account to link directly to other websites by posting a story with the 'swipe up' feature.
- **Tag:** a feature allowing a user to create a link back to the profile of the person mentioned.
- **Testimonial:** this can be online reviews posted on platforms such as websites or LinkedIn, typically in a professional context. Also referred to as 'Recommendations' and 'Endorsements'.

- **Thinspiration:** content that glorifies excessively skinny people, which may be shared with others.
- **TikTok:** one of the fastest growing social media platforms of all time, showing bitesize looping videos with music, that are tailored specifically to content that the user likes. Personally I find it highly addictive and can lost hours at a time on there.
- **Trending:** the most talked about topics and hashtags on a social media network, often seen on apps such as Twitter, inviting people to join the conversation.
- **Trigger Warning (TW):** this may be hash tagged in potentially upsetting posts such as those relating to mental health and making clear why (e.g TW: Sexual Assault). However, this might defeat the purpose of warning someone, as they could read it at the same time as the rest of the post. Alternatively, people could search #TW to read a stream of this content categorized together.
- **Troll:** a person creating controversy on social media, typically aiming to evoke negative reactions out of people. When a person is being 'trolled' they might receive lots of abuse at the same time, which could include very violent threats.
- **Tumblr:** a microblogging platform allowing users to share posts, often gearing towards communities with shared interests, which has been linked to anti-recovery communities.
- **Twitter:** a microblogging platform where users can share posts in 140 characters or less.
- **Twitch:** a live streaming social platform typically used by gamers to live stream their video games.
- **Unfollow:** the practice of literally unfollowing a person on social media. There are apps which can keep a person

updated with who's unfollowed them, which tend to be quite unhealthy!

- **Verified:** the issuing of a symbol such as a blue tick to give a user particular status, such as being a celebrity.
- **Video conferencing:** apps that allow video meetings to be held, such as Zoom and Microsoft Teams, or for those in a typically more casual context, Houseparty and Skype.
- **Viral:** a term used to describe an instance where a piece of content achieves noteworthy awareness.
- **Vlogging:** a video blog, with people who make them referred to as Vloggers.
- **YouTube:** a platform allowing users to create and watch videos, almost like an online television. People who create videos are typically referred to as YouTubers.
- **Webinar:** an online presentation hosted by an individual or a company, most commonly seen on Zoom. Social media apps such as Clubhouse have become popular recently in hosting live audio webinars on specific topics, facilitated by any user.
- **WhatsApp:** a messaging, phone and social media app allowing people to connect internationally. Messages can be 'archived' or made to disappear, and features can show whether a person is online or not.
- **What I eat in a day:** videos of a social media user showing what they claim to eat in an average day. This can obviously be inaccurate and result in normalised 'thinspiration', particularly if the user is glorified for their body type.

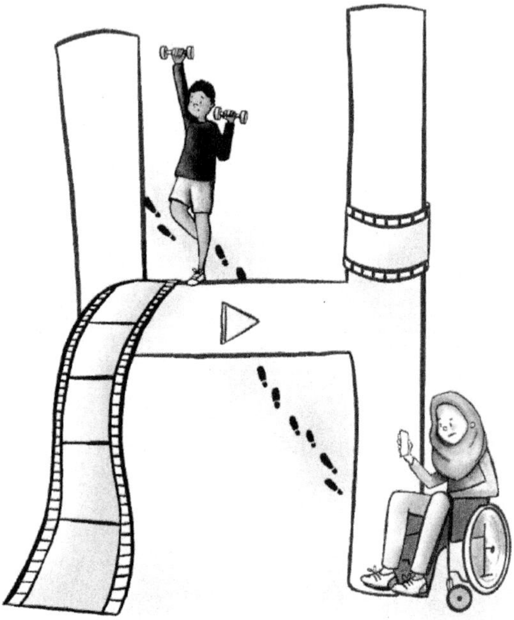

is for Health

H is for Health

Did you know?

- Targeted adverts on social media work by identifying your 'interest' in a topic. People with chronic illnesses have spoken about being targeted for adverts promising relief from their pain on social media.[19]

What does 'health' mean to you? When I was younger, the word 'healthy' was disgusting to me – it was like a barometer of being 'normal', which I equated with 'fat'. Now, it's become a impossible golden standard to reach, as technology gives me a daily update about how few steps I've taken.

When a model agency told me to lose 3 inches off my hips, as in 'D is for Disordered Eating', they said I could do this by just being 'healthy'. They said this meant 'not eating bread or chocolate' for a few weeks, and to 'exercise'. I was forced to pay for an expensive personal trainer, who told me it was literally impossible to get me to these measurements without me becoming very unwell.

She was right – I tried doing things 'healthily', but the weekly measuring ritual at my agency showed that just exercising and eating fruits and vegetables wasn't enough. I had to start starving myself and working out constantly, trying to study for my exams whilst walking on a treadmill. I became obsessed with calories, avoiding carbohydrates, and was often overwhelmed with trying to decipher food labels. Eventually I reached the measurements (to a round of applause) and went straight back up again the next week.

---

[19] Hannah Turner, 'I'm Chronically Ill & Social Media Algorithms Know It' (refinery29.com), 9 March 2022. Accessed 17 March 2022.

This is the world we're all living in, with an overload of information at our fingertips and a near-constant pressure to be perfect, both inside and out. Eating disorders and mental illnesses such as Bigorexia and Orthorexia are easily hidden behind being 'healthy'. Health has ironically become our society's new illness, as we obsess over trying to reach the glass ceiling of wellness.

This can feel an impossible world, because just like me as a teenage model, you can never be right. We're looking for the answers of how they 'should' be feeling in a world that's designed to manipulate us, losing connection with our own bodies and emotions. We're outsourcing their ability to understand our own wellbeing to technology, which will simply never let us feel good enough – it would be too good for our health to log off.

Physical health

As a child, I was told that sitting too close to the television would give me square eyes, but as an adult, I'm rarely more than an arm's length away from a screen. I used to fight about the half an hour of the dial-up internet I was allowed growing up, but these days, I've got to fight myself for half an hour away from it. These days, headphones blast electronically generated sound into my ears, drowning out my thoughts, and food delivery apps and video-conferencing software mean I never have to leave the house again.

What does this mean for the children growing up with this as 'normal' today? For those who attended school through laptops and were only allowed to go outside for one walk per day during the Covid-19 lockdown? Who weren't allowed to meet their friends, and who had to 'stay at home to save lives'? What does it mean for their eyesight, fitness levels, hearing, and vital organs?

It means they're getting worse – obesity rates are the highest they've ever been for all of us, and especially children. This might be surprising, given how much pressure there is to be 'healthy' and look a certain way online, but having pressure and access to information doesn't necessarily mean it will be used. In fact, just as I used to eat an entire box of chocolates on the way home from being measured as a model, it often has the opposite effect.

Information controls us

My phone can tell me how many steps I've taken, what my blood oxygen levels are, my heartbeat, my menstrual cycle, the number of calories I've consumed today, how well I slept last night, and how many times I've stood up today. I can find out the nutritional content of any food or drink item and access an endless stream of exercise videos.

These features can easily trick us into believing we should be able to manage the harms from the online world, but ultimately puts the responsibility on **us.** For example, you might be able to see how many hours you've been on your phone today, but then what do you do? How do you take control this when the technology is so addictive, as in 'A is for Algorithms'? If you could measure how much heroin you were taking in a day, would this give you any reassurance or control over the situation? How many hours is too many? Why don't social media companies publicly publish the screen time of different age groups, to give everybody the same understanding of what's happening to us as a society?

This overload of information can be presented to sell us the illusion of control, in a world that is simply uncontrollable. It shows us the problem and the solution, such as buying a smart watch for 'fitness', which could measure our steps and heart rate throughout the day. However, in a world where we can live entirely through a screen in the palm of our hand, a smart watch on our wrist isn't going to make us any more active. What it *will* do is make us even more accessible, during times we might not have been, such as in an exercise class, or whilst asleep!

It's an almost literal handcuff to social media, and we can easily ignore the reminders to 'stand up and focus', and instead on the notifications we receive from our friends showing up on our wrists.

These measurements ultimately become more yardsticks of failures, as in 'E is for Expectations', as they are simply more numbers to reach. Whether it's the number of calories consumed, steps taken, or the number of likes or followers received on social media in a day, these all become arbitrary figures that meaning can be attached to, such as being 'fit', 'healthy', 'productive', or 'successful'. They can become addictive in themselves, despite meaning nothing. A Diet Coke has less calories than a salad, but does this mean it's better for our health?

Features that allow a user to hide certain information, such as the number of likes they receive on posts or certain words from comments, simply provide a justification for continued use. Hiding problems doesn't make them go away, and the temptation of checking this information doesn't disappear just because it's been switched off. If anything, it could allow an even faker reality to be presented online – for example, the people I know with thousands of fake followers seem even more legitimate now, because their likes have been hidden.

Ultimately, this perpetuates the issues – the problem isn't a lack of information, but a manipulation of it. We don't need more information, but we need better information. Without it, users of social media are trapped in a cycle of beating themselves up for the harm they're experiencing online.

In a world where vulnerable young people are growing up in a world where social media has always existed, they experience these problems very differently to adults who grew up in the days of having dial-up internet connection and no phones. For many people, the simple and obvious answer will be to simply stop doing what is making us unhappy, but for many others, including children, this will be as impossible as simply deciding to stop breathing.

How health is manipulated online

There are a variety of ways health can be distorted by technology and social media, with the ultimate result of negatively impacting the way a person sees or feels about themselves.

For example:

- **Exercise videos**

Whilst moderate exercise is good for us, how do we stop doing a literal endless stream of free workouts for them to do in our bedrooms? Over-exercise can easily become a serious addiction and illness called Orthorexia, providing the illusion of control over our bodies, as in 'D is for Disordered Eating'.

- **Infographics and misinformation**

As in 'C is for Content', social media favours bitesize, easily relatable, and sharable content, which means important information can be miscommunicated. From Instagram posts comparing nutritional content and calories of different food items, to adverts by medical companies linking obesity to ADHD, it becomes very challenging to critically consider this information, and easy to relate to it.

- **Overload of information**

This is very relevant for search engines such as Google, which can show us an endless list of health-related information, leading to us possibly self-diagnosing ourselves with the worst possible scenario. By the time I was diagnosed with ADHD age 25, I'd convinced myself I had 10 different mental health conditions I'd seen on Google, and ADHD wasn't one of them!

This can also apply to features such as smart watches and habit tracking apps, that can provide us with data about ourselves we might never otherwise have known. This information might do nothing more than make us feel bad about ourselves (whilst giving technology providers extremely personal sensitive data), as we're still living in the same environments of using distracting technology, as in 'A is for Algorithms.'

- **Influencer diets**

Friends of mine became so obsessed with 'healthy' influencer diets that they only ate raw fruit and vegetables, becoming incredibly unwell. They eventually learned that the influencer they were copying was actually anorexic, and promoting a completely fake lifestyle.

Restrictive diets can easily be framed as moral obligations online, and even tied to certain beliefs, such as the ability to cure cancer. A previous friend of mine used to start her days with a garlic smoothie after reading about it online!

- **Health products such as 'vitamins'**

Social media influencers are often seen advertising 'health' products such as 'detox teas', 'vitamins', tablets, and powders. As in 'E is for Expectations', there's very limited oversight of adverts on social media, and these may often be completely misleading, such as the influencer not even using the product at all.

Even so, their audience may trust them implicitly, far more than they would a television advert by a company, for example. In the pursuit of looking or feeling as happy as their idols, they might buy these products, which can be extremely dangerous. In reality, these products may be the equivalent to buying drugs on the street – there's no way to know what's really in them, but this is normalised for people on social media, who might never otherwise be exposed to these 'magic fixes'.

- **Targeted adverts**

People may also be deliberately targeted by companies in relation to their health, by creating targeted adverts on platforms such as Facebook and Instagram to people with an 'interest in' a certain topic. So, if a persons' online activity showed them researching a certain health condition, such as ADHD, they might then be pestered with more information about this. I speak to at least one person a week who tells me they've diagnosed themselves with ADHD from social media!

This is arguably very unethical, as it's capitalising on peoples' health and related worries, and adverts may not be obvious.

- **Body positivity**

Although social media can be very empowering, it's ultimately always playing by the same rules of algorithms, as in 'C is for Content', objectifying our empowerment. For example, I previously posted a lot of body positivity content, comparing images of myself looking 'normal' in comparison to filtered or photoshopped versions of myself.

Even though I was objectively using social media in a 'healthy' way, I still felt the high of seeing these before and after version of myself, still subconsciously putting this 'perfect' version of myself out into the world. This is seen with trends such as those discussing eating disorders online, because it's still exposing people to the core content.

- **Fitness influencers**

What might start out as one person's fitness journey could easily spiral into an obsession if they build a community of like-minded followers. Whilst this might be great for motivation, it could also become unhealthy if a person is sharing content tailored to them that others may follow in the hope of being like them. Everybody is different, and food or exercise will impact us all differently.

This is especially relevant for children and teenagers, who have completely different metabolisms to adults, but who may idolize certain people. There's been trends of videos showing 'What I Eat In A Day' on apps such as TikTok which can be extremely harmful and act as 5-second diet guides, showing only the end result, which can easily be manipulated.

- **Trigger warnings**

Whilst it's brilliant that conversations about topics like mental health are happening more, it can also result in people possibly relating with content that may not actually be relevant to them in reality. For example, I know young children who diagnosed themselves with anxiety after watching YouTubers speak about being diagnosed.

Although 'trigger warnings' can be pasted onto certain online content, this puts responsibility on the viewer not to look at it, which may be too late given how subconsciously we read and process information. If anything, this content could become objectified in itself and become very confusing for a person who's receiving positive feedback about their negative experiences, possibly being manipulated to post more.

Staying healthy online

As someone who's experienced the never-ending 'health' treadmill, as distorted by social media, I believe the illnesses that can arise in relation to it are fundamentally emotional disorders, just like eating disorders. These could look like a person becoming obsessively anxious about health and exercise or believing there's something 'wrong' with them.

Again, in a world that feels uncontrollable, believing that you can at least control your own health – especially in the context of living through a global pandemic – might feel like a form of emotional release. For some, it might feel like a form of safety in their own bodies, and anyone talking to them about it may sound like the enemy, or as though they're dismissing their experiences.

It can be awful to experience, like you're trapped in a complicated prison of your own making, possibly resulting in compulsive behaviours that make you feel anxious without doing them, such as seeing your health data each day. I became so obsessed with calories and exercise that I would become angry with anyone trying to talk to me about it rationally, believing they didn't understand what I was experiencing and couldn't help as a result.

However, I probably would have benefited from speaking to someone who didn't judge me, who simply asked questions, and let me reach the answers for myself, such as a therapist or a coach. I coach people experiencing these issues and there's usually a fear underneath the behaviour, linking back to 'B is for Beauty'. Everything is interconnected.

As our society has become more technologically advanced, we've become more stressed, not less. When the world moved online during the pandemic, for example, the expectation was set that we'd be accessible online 24 hours a day, instead of leaving our laptops at work or school at 5pm, for example. The more 'time saving' advances we make, the less time we tend to have, because these technologies require managing. When they're being controlled by algorithms designed to make us use them more, we're actually wasting more of our time.

This is why the excess of information about health we can find online isn't healthy. Our ancestors weren't told how many steps they'd taken each day, the quality of their sleep, or the calories in their food, and they managed to survive and evolve. We have all of this knowledge, but don't know what to do with it. As our brains aren't designed to take in this much information, it's unsurprising that they start self-imploding.

It isn't natural for us to exercise all day, obsess over calories, or our health, which simply means that the underlying issues need attention to solve the external symptoms. When I changed model agencies, I started eating three proper meals a day, and exercising only because it felt good, instead of to look a certain way, because this is what naturally feels best for me. This is the difference between *feeling* healthy in your body and being *told* you're healthy. You aren't technology: only you know how you feel.

Tips

- Consider how you feel about your health: what does healthy mean to you?
- What would you score out of 10 your current fitness levels, sleep, diet, and energy levels?
- How healthy do you feel at the moment?
- Identify all of the health-related apps you use, and decide whether you want to continue using them in the same ways. How are they impacting your health?
- Take up new activities where you use your bodies in different ways, such as by going to yoga or joining a sports team.
- Remind yourself that you and the people in your life are healthy. It's easy to believe we're all in mortal danger online, but if you've got a problem, you'll know about it!
- Try meditating as regularly as you can, by simply taking a few minutes to check in with your body and observe how it feels. By getting to know what feels 'normal' or not, you'll be a much better health monitor than your phone!

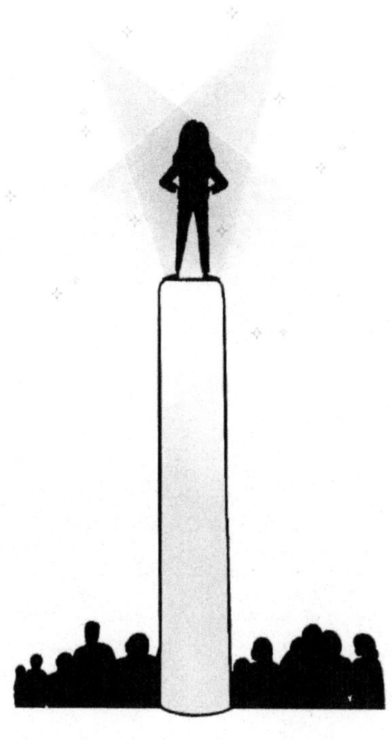

is for Influence

I is for Influence

Did you know?

- A 2019 study found there were 10 million fake Instagram accounts in the UK, and more than half of users here have bought followers, likes or comments. It's estimated 3 out of 10 influencers buy fake followers.[20]

When I was a teenager, it was possible to order your 'top' 8 friends on social media. We were less concerned with the opinions of strangers and more focused on our friends – the network we already had. I was obsessed with checking my friends' lists, seeing who liked me more or less than yesterday.

Today's social media is focused on the limitless global network we don't yet know. Though we don't rate our friends so obviously anymore, we do it by unspoken agreements of validation, such as by liking or commenting on each other's pictures. Today, connection can easily be replaced by 'influence' – leaving us feeling disconnected, lonely, and frustrated.

It can be easy to see wannabe influencers as attention-seeking, but when being liked equates to holding people's attention, this might feel like many peoples' only option. As in 'F is for Friendship', when friendships are being so publicly measured online, it can feel like a never-ending treadmill of maintaining a certain level of 'coolness' to stay relevant, both online and offline.

[20] Michael Baggs, 'Instagram: Why paying for followers and likes is bad news for real fans' - BBC News, 13 July 2019. Accessed 17 March 2022.

The difficulty is that we're in a world where influencers *are* being marketed as having the ultimate levels of happiness, love, friendship, and success in life. People with thousands of followers may appear happier than people with no followers, who might not post about their lives as much. If we believe a highlights reel of life formulated by the equation of followers = happiness, it's natural that we'd aim to become as popular as possible online.

As in 'E is for Expectations', the dangers of this are how impossible and fake it is. I experienced this myself, in believing that I just had to get a certain number of followers to be happy, which left me suicidal, blaming myself instead of the game I'd been manipulated into playing.

Fake fame

In the early days of Instagram, I signed with a 'talent' agency who didn't do much except repost my own modelling photos on their Instagram account, with over 20,000 followers. They kept saying I needed to grow my following to book jobs with them.

For a while, I beat myself up for not being able to suddenly get thousands of followers. I'd obsess over why I hadn't seen an increase in 'engagement' after this agency posted my photos, and started posting more photos of myself doing things like clubbing to get more followers, which didn't really make much difference!

This was until Instagram had a clean out of fake followers, which is proof that they can do this any time they want to. This agency's number of followers dropped dramatically by tens of thousands overnight. Suddenly their account had less than I did, and they admitted to buying followers, advising I do it too, giving me the link. Suddenly I had 10k followers at a cost of £50, feeling pretty pleased with myself – but this feeling disappeared as soon as I posted a photo. I felt like a huge fraud, and instantly wanted to remove the followers, but it was too late.

The anxiety and guilt ironically made me even more determined to get real followers, so I could somehow justify this or balance it out, but it was still as difficult as ever. It was only when I briefly dated someone famous that I started getting serious engagement. Every time he liked a photo of mine, I would get about 100 comments to update me. It was addictive and annoying, because clients had started asking me how many followers I had on Instagram at castings every day. I knew that this person liking my photos increased my status to them, even though it should have had literally no impact.

It wasn't long before I came across apps that provide fake likes and comments to keep up the high, as in 'V is for Validation'. These apps are incredibly dangerous and addictive. They're like influence filters – able to give you a rush of likes and validation, in the literal form of dopamine-hitting notifications. I loved my month of being adorned with 'free' likes and comments, and then found it very difficult to adjust back to reality when that month trial was over. The app would instead give a different number of surprise likes for free each day, and then you could buy them. It was like the slot machines found in casinos.

Within weeks, I was paying £10-20 per post for fake likes. I was addicted to Instagram and paying for it – literally. I wasn't alone, either – many of my fellow models were in this exact same situation. We were all under the impression that controlling our following on Instagram could give us a small measure of control over our careers, which we were literally powerless over. There's no way to get 'better' at modelling, because it all depends on the client of the day – but Instagram can give us a fake sense of control over it.

In the same way, social media gives us a fake sense of control over our own popularity levels. When you see someone with tens of thousands of followers, at least some are likely to be fake.

I also used to work for an app that gave models free gifts depending on how many followers they had. If you had less than 5k, you could get things like a free coffee at a café, 5-10k was a dinner, and over 10k was a free dinner for you and a guest, for example. I thought this was empowering, until I realised that somewhere along the way, someone was profiting. Models were unknowingly working for free, advertising companies on their Instagram accounts, and brands were paying for models with fake followers.

Another similar app popped up where models could go on holiday on a private jet or yacht, which sounds *amazing*, but in reality, someone else is paying for them to be there, who is likely expecting much more from them than simply advertising the holiday.

I finally learned the hard way that **there is no such thing as free**. By the age of 24, my Instagram account had photos of me on private jets, working for world-famous brands, and frolicking around a beach in a bikini, with over 15,000 followers. Every single experience required something in return, even if this was unspoken – from an Instagram post to pressure to sleep with someone.

I felt like I was trapped in this prison of a fake life, but couldn't get out of it, because it was what was allowing me to live. I moved to Byron Bay, the ultimate 'influencer' hub. It's a ridiculously beautiful place, but I couldn't enjoy it properly. I found myself waking up planning my Instagram posts, going to buy papayas to photograph on the beach, trying to find the sense of happiness that I looked like I had online. I felt like I had this imaginary audience, most of whom I knew didn't even exist, and I had to show up for them.

Social media can make you self-obsessed at the same time as viciously hating yourself. We forget that nobody cares what we do or don't post. No one would particularly care if the number of likes on my post suddenly stopped being the manufactured 150 and probably the more realistic 20 or 30. I see so many other models and 'influencers' with 50k, 100k, 200k etc followers, and only 50 likes on their photos. I know that it's fake, but what am I going to do, write to them and accuse them of having fake validation? Who really cares?

The only people who it may affect are those who survive financially from their online status, and the people who think their followers are real. I wasn't being paid by brands to promote them, but I was around this world every day, and saw how my friends were suddenly caught in complex webs of identity between who they were in real life, and who they were online. One could no longer be vegan, because she became very unwell, and received tens of *thousands* of hate messages as a result, asking for refunds of her cookbook. In contrast, other vegan 'influencers' I knew were simply lying about what they were eating online to their huge followings.

Fame doesn't equal happiness

I saw how lonely these famous people were, with only a couple of friends, despite having hundreds of thousands of followers. How they automatically assumed that people might be using them, and how they calculated whether someone was worthy of hanging out with by how many followers they had online.

Being an 'influencer' doesn't get any better the more followers you have, or more jobs you book – it gets worse. It locks you in to this identity that simply can't be everything you are, because it is a few squares on a virtual profile. It makes you dependent on the brands paying you, rather than being able to be authentic. You can never have enough followers – the need for more simply grows, and you just compare yourself to new standards. Having lots of followers made me feel awful about lying to the world and knowing I was making other people feel bad about themselves by projecting this image.

I ended up permanently deleting my account, as in 'Q is for Quitting', which was one of the best and most liberating decisions I've ever made. Ironically, I pitched this book to several book agents and publishers, who said I had to have over 10k followers on Instagram to sign with them! It was incredibly frustrating knowing that I could easily buy these followers and go back to them the next day, but I know how unhappy this made me. Besides, the entire point of this book is that you **do not need to have a following to be successful**!

Social media companies can detect fake followers and delete them, but they know that's what keeps people hooked. From a purely business perspective, having fake followers simply makes you seem more legitimate to real audiences, but they want to make money. The fakeness is just part of the sales tactics – if we think an account is already popular, we're more likely to follow it.

The difference is that you are *not a business*, as much as you might think of yourself as a CEO or boss or entrepreneur. You are a human being, who is naturally inclined to look at the tools of measuring 'success' by popularity that social media gives us. It's extremely difficult to go on social media without even subconsciously considering the numbers of likes or followers we see.

Just like the numbers on the scales, these numbers are meaningless – they don't necessarily translate into sales, or popularity, or stability. I knew Instagram 'models' with millions of followers who were terrible at brand partnerships, because the only people who followed them were men – and the brands wanted to access girls. Another photographer I know told me how he can't post the majority of his work, because he loses followers every time that he posts photos that aren't of a certain type of model in underwear.

As hard as it might feel, try to pull yourself out of this online world as much as you can, and remember how much of it isn't real. Don't allow social media to replace your ambitions and authenticity with its own – stick to what you love, and remember that social media really doesn't matter as much as we think it does. Everyone is far too worried about themselves!

If you're in the position I was, with fake followings and likes and so on, try to give yourself a break. Remember that the entire world of social media is distorted, from the algorithms that promote harmful content most, to the millions of fake bot followers. If you have bought followers, be kind to yourself – it's not your fault. Use all options there are to hide the number of likes you have on photos.

The best thing you could possibly do is take a break for a day, by deleting the app. Get rid of any apps that make you feel made about yourself, such as ones that give you 'likes'. Remember that NO ONE CARES about the number of likes or followers you have, but living in a way where you have to constantly live up to your own fake standards will make you anxious and stressed.

Tips

- I strongly advise against buying fake likes or followers, as this can lead to severe anxiety and shame building up in your head about it. If you already have and feel anxious, remember that no one really cares.

- When you see people with thousands of followers, likes, or comments, remember that they may be fake. Don't trust everything that you see online.

- Consider how much you care about your online following and engagement. Can you separate yourself from it?

- Avoid using any apps that tell you who has unfollowed you. You really do NOT need to know this, and it can send you off into spirals of insecurity! Try to avoid looking at these figures and remember that people may unfollow others for all sorts of reasons, including feeling insecure.

- Listen to yourself and your needs. Figure out what's missing from your life, and go do it – whether that's hanging out with friends, doing a hobby you enjoy, cooking a meal, whatever it is, just do it.

- Do whatever it is that you want to do **right now** (such as writing a book!) rather than waiting to have a certain number of followers, because they won't come.

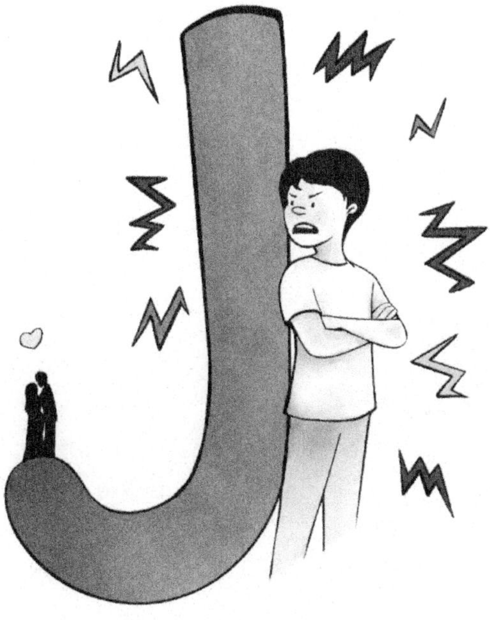

is for Jealousy

J is for Jealousy

Did you know?

- 58% of surveyed women said social media changed how others view them and how they view others, with only 14% having high levels of self-esteem, and 83% saying this is impacted negatively by social media.[21]

There was a girl in my primary school of whom I felt jealous. She was popular, and everyone seemed to think she was beautiful, whereas I was bullied for being ugly. She became my model, as I collected data on what she did and copied, whether that was washing my hair on certain school nights, or getting the same pencil case. Nothing changed.

This is the world we're all in now with social media, but on a hyper-level. We can see into the intimate details of people's lives we don't even know, people who we might imagine are happier than us. We can copy their morning routines, eat the same food, and buy the clothes they promote, but we don't become any happier.

We can have the same experiences as the people we admire, in a diluted form. We get to come along with them to A-List events, on their nights out, and on their holidays. It's like the virtual Neopet I had as a child, where I had to get on the computer to 'feed' it. We care deeply about these people, because we get to see different parts

---

[21] Alix Walker, 'Comparison culture is taking it's toll on our self-esteem', *Stylist Magazine*, accessed 17/3/22: www.stylist.co.uk/life/comparing-ourselves-to-others-comparison-culture-research-self-esteem-instagram-social-media-success-careers-fitness-relationships/345725?msclkid=4de1ab4ba5c411ecb9af9ae48f1695b7

of them, at the same time as wanting what they have. We think we know them, but we only know what they show us online.

In contrast, jealousy has always existed between us and people we know – it's a normal part of being human. The difference between 20 years ago and now in comparing your lawn or car to your neighbour's, is that now you can see inside their house. You can see what they're having for breakfast, what their opinions are, and inside their wardrobe. Rather than just buying a 'better' car than them, you might feel a drive to one up them in all sorts of ways – which usually involve spending money! The ironic thing is that they wouldn't even know this unless you posted it online.

Comparing ourselves to our peers online can be dangerous, as in 'C is for Content', because we might think this is more achievable than seeing a celebrity. For example, if your friend secretly bought 5000 followers, you might compare yourself and start copying them to try and get the same level of success, with no idea that these are fake. You might end up obsessing over that friend, becoming jealous of them and ending up not liking them anymore.

Social media gives us living, personalized highlights reels to compare ourselves to other people. The metrics and tools on these platforms distort our ability to simply connect with other people, because we're subconsciously comparing ourselves to how many followers or likes they have. Just because we might not post all of our achievements online, it doesn't mean we don't have any, but it can feel odd when we see how much validation other people get for this.

Ultimately, it boxes us into an uncomfortable place where we're competing with other people, who might not even know it.

Comparing ourselves to unreality

Subconsciously, no matter how much we think we love the people we look up to online, there's a part of us that's jealous of them too. There's a little part that's trying to figure out how we can be like them, how to get what they have, be who they are. There's no pot at the end of the rainbow: just look at how many celebrities have committed suicide. At the time of writing, *38* people have committed suicide after becoming famous from going on reality television. It's like we're living in a real-life version of the Hunger Games.

I know the feeling of insane jealousy, of weirdly hating someone you don't even know, but still finding yourself on their profile, scanning through their life, measuring yourself up against them. I feel paralysing comparison between me and other people doing similar work to me, as in 'P is for Perfectionism', wondering what the point of it is if I'm not as popular as they are. Even with people whose followers I know are mostly fake, I end up comparing myself in some way, wondering if I should have more. It's so frustrating to keep ending back up on their profiles, beating myself up for weirdly stalking them for no reason other than to compare myself.

The comparisons that social media provokes in us are incredibly dangerous. It infiltrates our relationships with other people, from our family to our friends, our daily experiences, everything about us. We hold ourselves up to these imaginary and completely fake standards, as in 'P is for Perfectionism', and try to fix ourselves in the hope of becoming better.

As in 'C is for Content', the danger of social media combined with the already existing problems of society such as 'size 0' models, is that it turns it into something even more impossible to achieve, because it simply does not exist. One study[22] found that Kim Kardashian's

---

[22] Jonathan Chadwick, 'Kim Kardashian's hourglass figure is more harmful for women's body image than Kate Moss' thin frame, study claims', *Mail Online*, 25 January 2022. Accessed 20 February 2022. www.dailymail.co.uk/sciencetech/article-10440489/Kim-Kardashians-hourglass-figure-harmful-body-image-study-says.html
Referencing the work of Sarah McComb and Jennifer S. Mills, 'The effect of physical appearance perfectionism and social comparison to thin-, slim-thick-, and fit-ideal Instagram imagery on young women's body image', *Research Gate*, March 2022.

'hourglass' figure is more harmful for body image than Kate Moss's thin frame, which may be because it appeals to a broader range of people. Just like me as a model being told to lose and gain weight in certain parts of my body as in 'E is for Eating', this is *impossible* to do.

Kim Kardashian hasn't even confirmed or denied having plastic surgery, leaving a glimmer of hope that just enough squats or sit ups might give someone her proportions. Even if you found her surgeon and had all the same procedures (if any), you wouldn't look like the airbrushed version of her, and you'd still be you, just possibly missing a few of your vital body parts.

Social media gives us this odd form of jealousy that isn't as obvious as wanting what someone else has got, such as me wanting to be the most popular girl in the school, but wanting to *be* someone else. This envy is based on comparisons, which leaves us beating ourselves up, because we think we *should* be able to look like our favourite influencers – after all, they've given us the steps to do it, such as buying their products!

This leads us to buy more and more things to feel better about ourselves. If we had no one to compare ourselves to, we'd have no reference for how our lives 'should' be but our own. We wouldn't be able to wake up and gorge ourselves on pictures of luxury yachts, idyllic beaches, plastic surgery, fame, and anything else we can imagine.

If all we had to compare ourselves to was a fleeting image on a billboard, that image would pass out of our minds, sooner or later. Compare this to the picture of Kendall Jenner 'behind the scenes' that caused a global wave of insecurity, which many girls told me was their new phone background as inspiration for them to stop eating.

---

www.researchgate.net/publication/357353298_The_effect_of_physical_appearance_perfectionism_and_social_comparison_to_thin-_slim-thick-_and_fit-ideal_Instagram_imagery_on_young_women's_body_image

When we've got someone to look up to, we can automatically compare ourselves, especially if this is playing out over a platform that is profiting from how much time we spend on it. On a platform where we can scroll past a photo of our face to see a famous celebrity next to us, our rational mind stops working. It doesn't register the celebrity as the equivalent of being on a giant billboard, but just compares that photo and number of likes to the one we've just seen of our own. It thinks we should be able to get the same, whereas most of us understand how unlikely it would be to end up on a billboard, having seen how brutal television programmes like 'America's Next Top Model' portray the industry to be.[23]

Whatever our insecurity is, we can seek it out on the internet and compare ourselves – and it finds us back. Targeted advertising seeks us out, showing us more of what we desire. It can show us more extreme versions, heighten our insecurities, driving us to buy products and hate ourselves. For example, if we wanted bigger lips, it might show us content focused solely on lips and fillers, causing us to believe our lips are unnaturally thin, even if we weren't surrounded by anyone in our real life who had fillers. These virtual worlds we compare ourselves to become our reality, and jealousy can take over our minds.

Reality

As in 'U is for Unreal', things are never as they seem online. I was previously very jealous of a girl who became friends with my friend, who seemed super successful and beautiful. When I ended up staying in her flat out of coincidence, I saw how she beat herself up daily for how much she weighed, and how much more she 'should' be doing. When I told her my story, as in 'E is for Eating', she said her life was changed, as she thought looking the way I did would make her happy.

---

[23] Someone I know went on this show in a different country, where the prize was to win a contract with a modelling agency. She was ALREADY WITH that modelling agency, who just wanted her to go on to boost her career – she came 2nd!

We ended up smashing her scales together in the street with a hammer!

It's important to remember that our brains are masters in creating stories about how much happier we'd be if we were different and tricking us into thinking we're alone in feeling this way. Everybody is going through the same experiences, and we all have the same basic experiences of being human, including all the stresses that come along with it, including insecurities and jealousy.

However, when we forget this, we can feel shame for feeling this way, imprisoning us in a cycle of negative thoughts. When we stop, accept, and notice what we're feeling, it can be giving us important messages about our own wants and needs. It's important to remember that jealousy is a normal human experience, that's being largely distorted by social media, and companies who profit from your insecurities.

Jealousy is a brilliant indicator of **what you want.** Often, it relates to something that we're feeling insecure about, and being curious about these feelings can help us understand what we might need to do in our own lives. We can't stop ourselves from comparing ourselves to others, but we can decide to approach this with kindness, both to the other person and ourselves.

By forcing ourselves out of the comparison world and into the real world, we can remind ourselves that 'success' generally comes after lots of rejection and failures, as in 'R is for Resilience'. The people I know who are the most objectively 'successful' in life only reached these places (such as Oxbridge universities) after being rejected multiple times and applying again – but this is what we don't see!

As you're human, you'll probably feel jealous at times, but by noticing this and have compassion for yourself and others, it can actually be very helpful in helping us to figure out what we need. Try to remember how social media is designed to distort these feelings, and take them offline.

Tips

- Consider who you're jealous of, and who you admire. What's the difference between these people?
- Identify the people whose profiles make you feel negatively about yourself, or those that you keep going onto, despite not liking or possibly even following them. Can you block or 'mute' these people? I used to have most of my friends muted on Instagram, as I hated feeling jealous of them!
- When do you compare yourself to others, and what do you do when that happens?
- Identify what's behind the feelings of jealousy or annoyance? What really makes you annoyed about a person or situation?
- If you compare yourself to someone, can you imagine them having all the same human experiences you have? From going to the toilet, to having relationship break ups, or experiencing the death of a loved on, how can you remind yourself that they're just as human as you are? A podcast called 'How to Fail' by Elizabeth Day is great for this!
- Can you feel gratitude to the person you're comparing yourself to, for helping you to realise what you're missing?
- Could you reach out to them for a chat, such as asking them to mentor you? The best way to stop putting someone in a pedestal is to get to know them in reality – we're all pretty much the same deep down, and all suffer with imposter syndrome!
- What would you change about you or your life, if you could wave a magic wand? Ask yourself 'what if' you had these things, how would your life change? What is the thing you genuinely want, behind the allure of fame, beauty, wealth and so on?

- Figure out what the corresponding action is to this in real life. For example, if you want to be more popular online because you feel lonely, can you join a new team or group meeting, or reach out to people in your life to meet up? If it's because there's something you're feeling scared to do, can you push yourself to just do it?

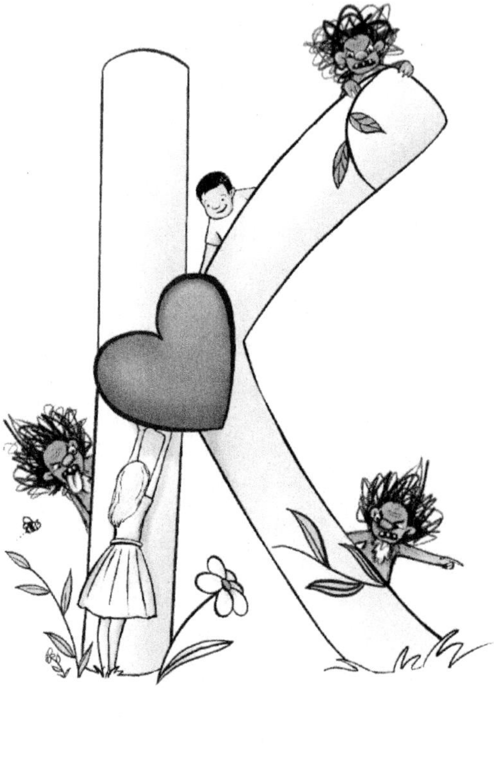

is for Kindness

K is for Kindness

Did you know?

- If something has been shared online 20 times in a row, it's 10 times more likely to contain nudity, violence, hate speech, or misinformation, than a post that's not been shared at all.[24]

Social media can easily bring out the worst in us, especially when its sole motivation is to keep us on the platform, as in 'A is for Algorithms'. It gives us anonymity to hide behind, provokes our insecurities, makes us act impulsively, and can easily make us forget that we're engaging with or about real human beings, who come with all the same complex feelings and insecurities that we do. Behind a screen, we're given a fake sense of control and power that we might not feel in real life, which can easily become an addiction in itself.

We're also much more likely to follow and be followed by people who think like us, because we like having what we believe confirmed – in other words, being right. When we see something that challenges this, we can easily want to regain this sense of control by being unkind, to try and make ourselves feel better.

The saddest thing about this, is that nobody wins. It doesn't feel good to be horrible to others, because we know what it feels like to be unhappy. All humans have empathy, the ability to understand and share the feelings of other, and without this, we lose the essence of being human – the ability to build social connections. As in 'A is for Algorithms', we're wired to seek out potential threats and negativity, so we will naturally focus on one negative comment more than 100

---

[24] 'The Facebook Files: A Wall Street Journal Investigation', accessed 20 February 2022. www.wsj.com/articles/the-facebook-files-11631713039

positive ones, severely impacting our self-esteem. Seeking this confirmation of the negative beliefs we may have about ourselves, such as feeling ugly, can also become an addiction of sorts online, by searching for negative comments.

When we're around other people, we subconsciously pick up on subtle body language and reflect this to each other, such as maintaining eye contact. Our bodies also release 'feel good' hormones like oxytocin, as we've evolved to need connection for the survival of humanity. When we do this through a screen, we don't get these benefits. We can easily check our emails during a zoom meeting, text other people when we're on the phone, or ignore text messages that we don't want to reply to.

The internet can easily make us behave in ways we wouldn't in real life, because we can't see the people we're talking to. In response to feeling ashamed of our behaviour, we may try to make ourselves feel better by proving ourselves to be right, leading to the same pattern, until we're completely detached from ourselves and our sense of shame. It sets the new standard for what we think is 'normal' behaviour, but no matter how much we can try to justify it to ourselves, being unkind is never going to make us happy, even if everybody else seems to be doing it too.

Trolling

Being bullied to your face is an odd experience. At school, kids called me ugly, laughed at my 'yellow' skin, and called me a transvestite for being tall, but I didn't know what I was meant to do with this information, as these were things that I obviously had no control over. A decade later, I received near-daily hateful public messages from an ex-boyfriend online. Blocking him made me feel momentarily in control, but then he'd just make a new anonymous profile.

The lack of control I felt over when these messages would come, where they'd appear, and what they'd say, sent me spiralling into constant anxiety, obsessing over what could happen next. At one point, I was too scared to go outside in case he sprayed acid in my face, as I'd read about in the news. I was in a constant state of 'fight or flight' mode, checking my phone throughout the day to see whether he'd messaged. This quickly became an addiction, where I'd almost feel a sense of relief if he had messaged, despite it being horrible to read, like a bizarre form of self-harm.

Whereas I felt lonely and powerless at school, social media gave me a self-destructive form of fighting back by trying to get control in this way. I started posting photos of me 'living my best life' to try and prove him wrong, which unsurprisingly, only made his messages more abusive. It also made me feel worse, as I played out this out in real life, such as posting photos of dates with people I didn't even like to get the hit of feeling in control by provoking more abuse on my terms, instead of his.

I started to actively seek the messages out, because they reaffirmed my belief that I was a terrible person, driving me into a dark depression. It reached the point where if he didn't message me one day on a new profile, I'd unblock him, and he'd immediately start again, demanding that I re-block him. The lines became blurred, but by reaching this point, at I felt like at least I deserved his hate – I could understand it, unlike when I was bullied at school.

He probably looked utterly unhinged to the people in his life, yet neither of us could stop this self-destructive cycle. It was an addiction, kept alive by Instagram, continuing even after I'd moved to the other side of the world. Obviously, none of this gave me any sense of real control, leading to me feeling like ending my life was the only way it would ever end.

The shame of feeling responsible for the abuse I was receiving stopped me from getting help for this, which is why it played out so unhealthily as I tried to handle it by myself. Eventually, I broke free by deleting my entire Instagram account and responding to any further messages to say they'd be referred onto the police, but it was one of the hardest things I've ever overcome.

Trolling is when online posts are made with the deliberate aim of upsetting someone. UK law doesn't have a legal definition of bullying, and it's not against the law by itself, even in a formal setting such as a workplace. Even if there was, the internet offers us a wild west of anonymous profiles and manipulations of our behaviour, leading us to blame ourselves.

It's easy to tell someone to just 'ignore it', but this can be impossible when we're using platforms designed to give us other people's opinions about us – that's the whole point. Telling someone to ignore an abusive comment reaffirming their own deep insecurities is like telling someone not to feel pain when they're punched in the face – it's impossible. Social media can easily drag us into these virtual battlefields, making us behave in ways we don't understand and turning us into people we no longer recognise.

Being kind doesn't typically get as much attention online as being angry, which keeps us returning to the platform – we're being provoked. Not by the person whose opinions we disagree with, but by the platforms that engineer us to share, retweet, and comment on their opinions. When we adopt these personalities online, sooner or later, they become us in real life too. When we're unkind to others, we're also being unkind to ourselves

Cancel Culture

In the last few years, cancelling people has become an online trend – essentially, making them not relevant, often by ending their career. For me, this feels like socially acceptable and normalized trolling on a mass scale. Whereas gossip magazines have always blasted the mistakes of celebrities on their front pages, today, we've all become both the editors and potential celebrities in a non-stop culture of moral outrage. Any one of us could find ourselves being publicly shamed for reasons outside of our control, with this unpredictability and fear of being cancelled keeping us anxiously trying to show we're not bad people, instead cramming ourselves into the editors' room.

Whilst we could have previously chosen not to read gossip magazines, today, we're used to reading news updates 24 hours a day on social media platforms. There's no guidebook on how to avoid being cancelled, or what the right or wrong thing to say is, as our society changes so quickly. As nobody wants to risk being virtually killed and feeling like they're hated by the world, we can all flock to social media or news platforms to try and keep up to date with how we 'should' be acting. Just look at the top comments under any news article – usually, they tend to all be similar.

The problem with this is that we've normalized judging other people we don't even know, often in extreme ways. We seek out gossip magazines now like religious guidance, with the new obligation of having to display our own allegiance to avoid being in them ourselves. When we 'cancel' human beings, we're effectively saying it's justified for a person to be bullied and pushed to the point of not even being able to make an income to survive. As in 'Y is for Your Truth', this can also often come from bite-size content on the internet, presented to us only in a way that will automatically trigger our outrage, rather than showing a balanced opinion.

Often, the bullying comes in forms that are far worse than simply being ignored – on the contrary, the person is usually subject to unimaginable amounts of online hate and threats about their or their loved ones' personal safety. The law is the foundation of our society, and although it's not perfect, if we take it into our own hands then we risk living in a world with no co-operation, organisation, or basic respect between different people – we risk losing our humanity.

After I published *the Model Manifesto,* a model agency owner called me up crying. One of her models had posted all over social media to 'cancel' her agency, even creating a new dedicated account. She was angry that she hadn't been paid, but as the agency owner explained to me, the client hadn't paid either, meaning she didn't have the money to pay her. I realised how hard it must be to be in that position – something I'd not really considered before. We all have complex reasons for the way we are.

We ended up having separate conversations with the model to calm her down. She'd been sent legal letters to warn her about the risk of being sued for defamation, but this just made her worse. It was only by having a genuine conversation she could understand the other perspective and stop wanting to destroy this woman's entire livelihood. I've had several conversations like this over the last few years, with people becoming intensely angry and wanting retribution via social media.

Just like trolling, cancelling someone only leaves you worse off. The anger spiral that can emerge from hate, wanting revenge, to seek justice yourself, or change a flawed system, can easily destroy you. It can take over your mind, becoming an obsession, and a distraction from yourself. Judging other people also imprisons you from being able to be yourself out of fear that you may accidentally make a mistake, as in 'R is for Resilience'.

It's a waste of energy trying to bring someone else down, change their beliefs, or prove yourself to be right – you'll never know when you're done. People are neither all bad nor all good. We all have shades of light and dark within us, but social media stops us from being able to see that.

I wrote *the Model Manifesto* to provide a solution to exploitation, instead of trying to bring down particular people. It took me many experiences of becoming extremely unwell through becoming so obsessed with revenge to get to this point, but I have never, ever regretted forgiving as best I can and walking away. Your peace of mind and sanity is worth so much more than trying to make things right, all by yourself. There will never be any better feeling than the freedom to be happy on your own terms, which is really all we're really seeking when we're trying to prove ourselves online, as in 'V is for Validation'.

To be kind to others, start with yourself. Simply take the time each day to figure out what makes you happy, and do that, instead of scrolling away on autopilot. When we're happy in ourselves, it's much harder for the opinions of other people to upset us. When we do things that make us feel good, like seeing people we care about in real life, we're able to control our own levels of happiness in a positive and productive way.

Being kind to other people also has been proven to make us feel happier. If you're feeling stuck, start volunteering. Try to spot opportunities for kindness in real life and take them – be the change you want to see in the world.

Tips

- Consider how you feel about yourself: do you like yourself? Would you want to be friends with you? Why or why not?
- How do you feel about people who've been 'cancelled'? Do you believe they should die, or never work again? How does thinking this make you feel? Can you imagine a world in which they were driven to act the way they did, such as by having a terrible childhood or needing help? How does this change things?
- If you're subject to any online bullying or unkindness, such as negative comments, how do you react? I'd strongly advise deleting and blocking anyone who is negative towards you, rather than getting into an argument. It's very difficult to change peoples' minds, especially online, and there will always be people seeking to bring others down because of their own unhappiness, as in 'J is for Jealousy', but this doesn't mean you have to see it.

- If you're feeling insecure, what do you do to feel better? Can you identify something that isn't related to social media to feel better, such as a yoga class or writing in a journal?

- Remember that social media can amplify and distort our negative feelings, so try to use it only when you are feeling confident and happy in yourself.

- Try to figure out what you feel insecure or angry about, and how you can process this away from social media, such as writing a book like this one!

- Speak to someone in an environment where you don't have to fear being judged, such as a therapist.

- If anyone sends you messages that make you feel uncomfortable after blocking them, I'd strongly recommend going straight to the police. This might feel drastic, but imagine if it was someone outside your house!

- If you've noticed patterns of behaviour you don't want to be doing, try taking a break from social media, as in 'Q is for Quitting'.

- Try to slow down your response levels and pause before posting something online, as in 'C is for Content'. Ask yourself what your underlying intention is behind this.

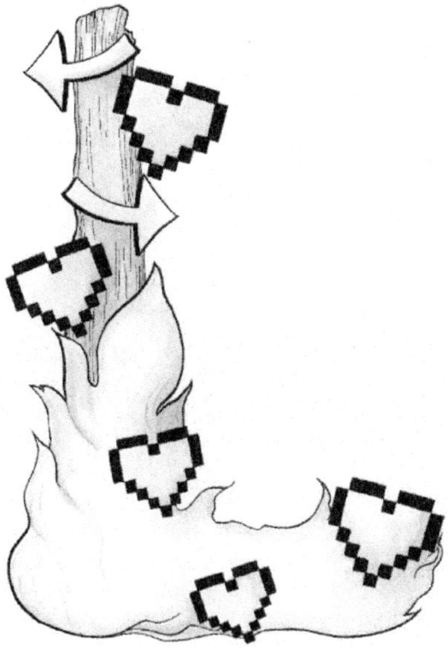

is for Love

L is for Love

Did you know?

- Almost 1 in 2 marriages end in divorce – and this is *6 times* more likely if you met your partner online.[25]

If you want to feel instantly bad about yourself, try setting up a profile on a dating app. There's nothing quite like trying to advertise yourself to your potential soulmate by thinking of clever answers to prompts like, 'How My Mother Would Describe Me', and 5 carefully selected photographs.

Using a dating app is like playing a video game, but with the potential of meeting someone in real life at the end of it, a dopamine thrill that's impossible to beat, because it's unpredictable. It can be a demoralizing and addictive experience, controlled by an algorithm feeding directly off our need for validation, comparisons with other people around us and fears of being alone.

We're invited to float in a sea of limitless profiles, waiting for someone to throw us a lifeline and save us. We might be out there for what feels like such a long time, that we're willing to settle for birds dropping sticks into the water. Our brains can work with this – we can turn the sticks into yachts, the birds into the loves of our life – before reality hits again, plunging us back into drowning.

This is because the house always wins, as we struggle to settle for anything less than the impossible ideal of perfection we've created in our minds. Dating apps, as much as they may portray themselves as

---

[25] Microsoft Word - Draft MF note - Where did you meet your spouse.doc (marriagefoundation.org.uk)

benevolent matchmakers, are corporations making huge amounts of profits from our insecurities.

The apps amplify our society's Disney-narrative that the point of life is to fall in love and fall happily ever after, despite this rarely being the case in reality. Love is a very powerful tool for capitalism, often underlying why we want to be 'beautiful', as in 'B is for Beauty'.

Dating allows us to present ourselves as we'd *like* to be and perceive people as we want them to be. It's only when we're past the novelty stage, that we're forced to see how people are in reality, but apps fast-forward this process. It's much easier to pretend to be someone else online than it is in person, like when I had a month-long 'relationship' over text, before meeting the person and realising I had a completely different idea of them in my head. I'd even get into full blown relationships with people believing this narrative, only being confronted with the truth months down the line.

This can result in a rollercoaster of emotions, where we're having entire relationships in our heads, putting huge amounts of energy into something that doesn't exist in reality. When it doesn't work, the easy answer is to blame ourselves.

People have become replaceable, especially when they've got annoyingly human habits, such as not doing exactly what you want to do on the weekend. If you've got the temptation of an entire world of other people in the palm of your hand, how do you ever settle for the reality of imperfection? When I started using dating apps, I was constantly upgrading and replacing people, which left me pulling myself apart and creating new identities every month. I was addicted to dating, and couldn't have a healthy relationship, because I was so used to having someone new. Human relationships are messy and complicated, requiring work and continuous effort, but apps can disguise this and make us think it should simply be easy, because we've 'matched' with someone that appears to like us back.

Commodifying love

As in 'A is for Algorithms', when something is free, you are the product. Dating apps make money from your attention, with lots of features that equate to just one extra turn on the gambling machine. For example, by charging extra to 'swipe' more than a limited number per day, after tantalizingly showing you a picture of someone you find very attractive. It's easy to forget that these algorithms have understood how to sell you what you want and are optimized to make you spend money or keep swiping.

For example, one app kept showing me people who were under 5'11 (my one requirement as I'm insecure about being so tall), leading to me to pay for the ability to apply this filter. Others might deliberately limit the number of matches you get, so that you pay to have a promoted profile.

I used to be part of an invite-only dating app called Raya, where scores of models, celebrities and 'influencers' would appear, basically making it like another version of Instagram. I met one person from there, where we acknowledged how ridiculous it was that we were paying to be part of an exclusive dating club based off how many Instagram followers we had – the whole thing felt fake, weird, and shameful.

When we're in control of how we use them, dating apps open the possibility of connections much wider than waiting for a new person to move into your village, or join your workplace, like our grandparents had to. However, they need to be used carefully, as they encourage us to gamble on genuine human connection, playing with peoples' emotions and lives – and our own.

They can easily make us think there is a problem with us, when actually, there's a problem with any system that is profiting from exploiting our loneliness. It's easy to forget that the apps that connect us, also control us, and that they profit from our insecurities, despite being 'free' to use.

Dating Slot Machines

Level 1: creating a profile that doesn't make you feel like a loser & judging others

It's very difficult to package yourself up into a profile of neat Q&A's and pictures you 'might find on my grandma's fridge'. I'd often use professional modelling pictures to get more likes, making me feel insecure about meeting people in real life as the non-professionally made up or photoshopped human being I am, as in 'E is for Expectations'. I even got banned from an app once for apparently using fake photographs!

Other people may not have lots of 'go-to' photos to use for dating apps, and the temptation to highlight what we'd *like* to be us, rather than what is actually us, is very strong, making us feel insecure.

There's the initial swiping, our subconscious judgements manufactured into a game of casting for our future soulmate by swiping right or left, making us the judges of our own reality shows. When the notifications of likes or matches pop up on our screen, they activate our brains like dollar signs on slot machines, a signal of potentially winning the jackpot.

Our expectations of how much interaction we should be getting at this level can make us feel really bad about ourselves. We might have high standards of others, but not receive many likes in return, or compare ourselves to our friends' levels of engagement. I liked virtually everyone, just to get the highs of the matches, especially if I was feeling insecure! This led to me feeling obligated to respond to and meet people I wasn't even attracted to – not the best start for a relationship!

Level 2: matching with someone who looks like they could possibly be our soul mate

Once we've matched with someone we vaguely like, this can easily spiral us into obsession over someone we don't even know, stalking them on the internet, planning out our future with them, and very possibly accidentally liking their social media posts from years ago (as I have done, many times). The excitement of matching with your potential *future soul mate* plunges you onto the next level of virtually 'getting to know' them, which is also highly fast-forwarded in the online world.

This might come with texts, phone calls, video chats, voice notes, and more. There's no clear etiquette of how often or when to text someone, but your brain might be feeding itself on 24-hour daydreaming about them. It's very easy to have a full-blown relationship with someone in this way, which I'd often refer to as just having 'someone to text'.

Level 3: meeting in real life

By this point, you might have created the perfect narrative to fit your date. Alcohol or infatuation can help smooth over any bumps during the short amount of time you spend together in reality. We've often invested a lot in a person by this point, making it very tempting to ignore our gut instincts in the hope of winning the game and getting off the apps. When I started out on the apps, I'd often suggest a shot of tequila at the start of my first dates – which was a TERRIBLE idea!

There's also the agony of figuring out what dates to do, and how to pay for them. Dating can be expensive and can feel like it comes with all sorts of obligations. Meeting someone you realise you're not attracted to, and watching them order half the menu in an expensive restaurant can be very anxiety inducing! After lots of trial and error, I decided to keep dates to free, daytime activities, not including alcohol, which helped me understand if I actually liked someone enough to hang out with them, with no other distractions.

Level 4: 'seeing' each other

If your date goes well, maybe there'll be more. Not knowing of whether your potential soulmate is also going on dates with other people, or whether they'll text you back within 5 hours, can be quite hellish. Many times, I have acted completely erratically during this time, after a brilliant date and expecting that the other person should immediately start texting me throughout the day.

We often have nothing to compare our experiences on dating apps to, and some people might be using them much more than we are. As in 'K is for Kindness', technology can also make us less compassionate towards others, and we might end up being 'ghosted' – or in other words, completely ignored by someone we're talking to. This is a horrible thing to experience, and can leave you questioning everything, trying to figure out what went wrong. In reality, the person might just have been on 5 dates that week!

Level 5: reality – return to 'Level 1' and try again!

If all goes well, maybe you'll reach the 'winning' point, whatever that is for you. For me, this was when we agreed to be 'exclusive'. At this point, the dopamine, which simply has the job of 'seeking' pleasure, wears off, just like a drug. For me, the second I got into an official relationship and reality began to set in, the thrill of not knowing what would happen would wear off. It felt completely out of my control, but I'd start to *not* like the person as soon as they committed to liking me, and I'd unconsciously search for a reason to break things off.

I usually blamed myself, feeling like a terrible person for hurting someone in this way, before getting straight back on the apps to do it all over again in the hope of making myself feel better. It didn't help that I'd often be spotted by them or their friends days later on the apps, proving that I didn't need as much 'alone time' as I'd said – but I simply *could not control it.* The worse I felt about myself, the more hooked I became to seeking redemption, and repeating it all over again, as in 'V is for Validation'.

After using dating apps for a while, you begin to see the same faces. They become depressing vortexes of souls looking for souls, literally being sold the illusion of their perfect soulmate, with just one more swipe. Apps make it make it near impossible to get into a healthy relationship without always wondering who else is lying in wait, distorting our view of what healthy relationships are: work. If we're dating out of loneliness, we will end up in unhappy relationships, feeling more alone than before.

This is what I've learned about dating: **you have to actually like the person for who they are.** Your life has to be better with them in it, than with them not in it. Whilst nobody is perfect, and there will always be little parts of the person you're dating you might want to change slightly, you will *choose them.* Dating apps sell us this story that we should be dating someone who's perfect for us in every way, but the reality is, that real relationships take effort and work.

Until we find someone who we like enough to put that effort in for, I recommend choosing to be alone. You do not need another human being to complete you, and being lonely is very different to be alone – not comparing yourself to other couples, but simply doing what makes you happy in life. Just like other social media platforms, dating apps in themselves aren't inherently bad, and seem to be the main way people meet each other today, but it's extremely important to stay conscious of your self-esteem and motivations whilst using these apps.

If you get sucked into the dating app dilemma, remember that you are working against the world's top behavioural engineers. Try to remember that being alone and happy is much better than being with the wrong person, and that the online world is largely dictated by algorithms.

Instead of trying to change yourself to fit it, be more of yourself in the real world. Do the things you enjoy, call people you love, see friends, get a massage, go to a yoga class – the world is filled with opportunities for happiness, and they don't all have to rely on finding your soulmate. Above all, remember that your relationship status says nothing about your worth as a person. You are 100% whole and loved, exactly as you are.

Tips

- If you use dating apps, how do you find this? How much time do you spend on them a day? When are you most likely to use them?

- Try to identify boundaries you could put in place for using these apps, such as deleting them from your home screen, or only using them at certain times. It may be helpful to identify what makes you feel insecure or anxious about dating apps, such as waiting for responses to text messages, and taking corresponding action, such as silencing notifications.

- Remember to be very careful with using dating apps and meeting people from the internet, who might not be who they say they are. Although it's become normalized to meet up with strangers, try to always meet them in a public place and avoid giving out your personal information.

- Identify why you're using dating apps – is it for a long term relationship? By being clear about what you're looking for, you can avoid wasting your time. If you're looking for social connections, can you look for an activity to do in real life that you enjoy instead, such as volunteering?

- Identify what you want from a relationship in general – what type of person do you want to meet? What are your interests and hobbies? What are your 'deal breakers' for a relationship?

- If you can, try to shift any online relationships into the real world as soon as possible, so you can determine whether you actually like this person, instead of texting each other updates about your days. At the same time, slow down the dating process as much as you can, and try to enjoy getting to know each other without the pressure of a relationship.

- Listen to yourself and how you feel, rather than trying to shoehorn yourself into relationships with people just because they meet a list of arbitrary requirements, or seem 'nice enough'.

- Try to avoid spending money on dating apps, if you can. This can lead to unconscious spending and addictive behaviours, as in 'M is for Money'.

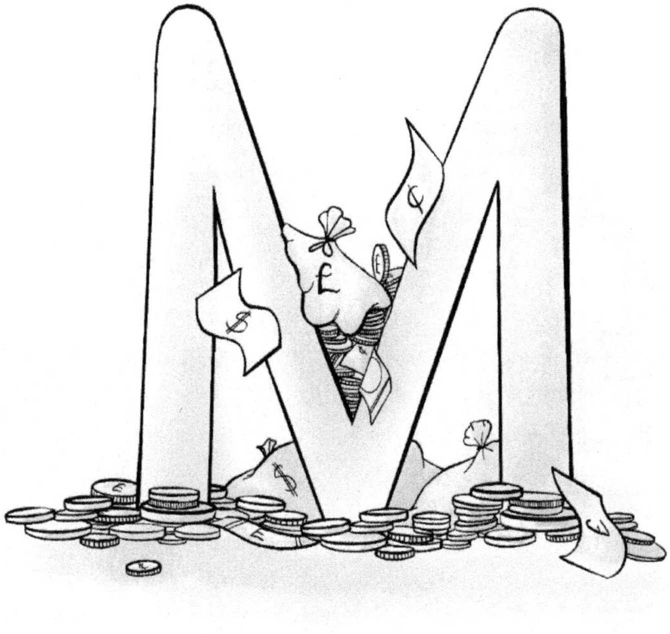

is for Money

M is for Money

Did you know?

- The Advertising Standards Authority's 2021 influencer monitoring report found that only 35% of Instagram advertising posts were compliant with ASA rules. [26]

Have you ever wondered why social media platforms like Facebook are free to use, whereas others charge money? It's because you are the product. The only industries that call their customers users are drugs, and technology. You are the user, and your attention is what's for sale.

If you had to pay £5 every time you went on your favourite social media platform, would this change how you used it? Technology companies are not benevolent charities, and whilst many of us may not care that someone like Mark Zuckerberg would care about what we do on the internet, we should.

As in 'A is for Algorithms', the more information social media companies can collect about users, the more accurate predictions they can make about our behaviour. Whilst some of these predictions might be useful, such as suggesting which movie we might enjoy watching next, others might be very much against what we want, such as influencing who we vote for in an election.

The ultimate problem with this is that the users are not the end customer – whoever is paying for our information is, but we don't necessarily know who they are. In contrast, they know more about us

---

[26] Advertising Standards Agency, 'Influencer Ad Disclosure on Social Media', 2021, accessed 17/3/22: www.asa.org.uk/static/dd740667-6fe0-4fa7-80de3e4598417912/Influencer-Monitoring-Report-March2021.pdf

than we might know about ourselves, understanding how to keep us using addictive products, spending more money, and behaving as intended. In this way, we are the 'user', hooked into a cycle that is very challenging to break out of, especially when we don't even realise that we're in it. Social media platforms can also create a strong sense of trusting what we see on there, as in 'E is for Expectations', making us vulnerable to people who want to exploit us, such as scamming us financially. When this happens online, it can be very difficult to get help from the platforms responsible for facilitating this.

Impulsivity

Most days during the first Covid-19 lockdown, I received surprises in the post. These weren't from admirers, but myself - because I'd often forgotten even ordering something in the first place. I'd see something, justify it in my head (usually along the line of not being able to go out and spend money due to the lockdown), and buy it. I was surrounded by junk and things I didn't need, but the effort of returning any of it far outweighed the high of receiving it, so I just kept them.

One of the major challenges in having ADHD is impulsivity, which can become very serious in a financial context. As my brain is constantly rushing around, I can often find myself ordering things without thinking it through properly – so I have to take additional steps, like regularly doing a 'subscription clear-out', and recording how much money I spend each week, in order to stay on top of my spending.

In contrast to this, the online world wants us to spend money as seamlessly as possible, whether we have ADHD or not. The less time we have to think about what we're doing, such as getting out a credit card and remembering a password, the more impulsive we are, making it more likely that we follow through with our purchase. Compare how easy it is to press a button and have something delivered to your house a few hours later, with the stress of returning it. The thought of finding a printer, sorting out the various return labels, sourcing packaging, going to the post office, standing in a queue and sending off a package to return is just not something my brain will engage in.

Instead, the packages will sit on the side for days on end, gathering dust. This is the world we're all in now, where we can literally order as seamlessly as speaking the words out loud to a smart device listening to us. The potential for us to be manipulated can be significant here – we're unable to see different options and have to trust what we're being told by technology. To think for ourselves takes more effort.

This is making us more and more used to a quick, impulsive way of spending money, making it harder to adapt to processes that require sustained mental effort on boring and unstimulating tasks, like being placed on hold. Fast fashion fuels this impulsive, novelty-driven world, with clothes so cheap to buy that it seems pointless to spend the money and time in returning them.

Another hallmark of ADHD is a challenge in 'delayed gratification' – as in, if we want something, we want it *now.* We don't want to wait until payday. 'Buy Now, Pay Later' companies have popped up everywhere, creating habits in us of getting into 'ok' debt, as an online payment is spread out over a longer period for a minimal cost. During Fashion Week a few years ago, a company like this sponsored a show I went to see, which I thought was quite bizarre, as models were dressed up in t-shirts with their name. However, today, this company is now featured on most e-commerce websites, fostering impulsive spending, debt, and addiction.

Whilst spreading the cost of 1 new t-shirt out over 6 months might seem manageable, 6, or 60, new t-shirts might be less so. The new habits that are quickly becoming ingrained in us to buy now, and figure out paying later, make us more prone to buying things we don't need. The quicker and easier something is to have, the less we appreciate it, and our dopamine neurotransmitters are on the hunt for the next thing.

The 'subscription' model of payments is also problematic in terms of impulsively signing up to free trials and forgetting about them. They work by making signing up seamlessly easy and cancelling virtually impossible. I know a woman who's had a newspaper subscription payment leaving her account for *years* because she can't figure out how to cancel it, despite never receiving the paper as it must have the wrong address!

I've lost track of how many different emails and passwords I've used for free trials, which is a nightmare in trying to cancel them. Similarly, to organising returns we've ordered, the process of cancelling can be so bureaucratic that we just give up, especially for things that seem like a 'small' cost. When we add this up, it might be hundreds of pounds a year!

This all relates to unconscious spending – where we're buying things so automatically and quickly that we don't even recognise what's happening. Buying things online may feel no different to clicking a button or sending an email to our brains, but it has a very real difference to our bank accounts. New technology such as 'smart speakers' can both pick up on more information about what we might be willing to spend money on and provide us new, and even easier ways of shopping.

Hidden adverts

Whilst we can recognise e-commerce websites as places we'd spend money, we don't have such obvious expectations with social media. As in 'O is for Objectification', The lines are extremely blurred between what we're promoting and why, and who's profiting – for example, fashion brands account for over 31% of total interactions on Instagram.[27]

Social media content is user generated, and whilst big companies might have to have returns policies and abide by consumer laws, the murky world of social media is a completely new marketplace – literally. For example, 'explore' pages on Instagram present to us exactly the type of products we might like, enabling us to purchase with a simple tap of the finger. These pages are formatted very similarly to the usual scrolling page, making it very difficult to tell the difference between the different types of content we're being shown.

These platforms can also make us believe that products are presented in a more realistic way than by companies on their websites, but the opposite is often true. For example, people selling diet products whilst editing their photos to appear thinner, who claim it's because of this product, have very little legal oversight over whether they're telling the truth. Social media sells us an entire lifestyle, and it's extremely difficult to regulate or quantify this. For example, although Kendall Jenner was fined $90,000 for promoting a festival that didn't happen, she was reportedly paid $250,000 for this post.[28]

Whereas a 'traditional' mascara advertisement would not legally be able to use fake eyelashes, there's nothing to prevent this from happening by an 'influencer' who is being paid to promote some mascara. They might even use a filter that gives them digitally enhanced eyelashes. How about if the filter simply changed their skin, or the lighting around them?

---

[27] 'Fashion accounts for the dominant share of Instagram interactions, but e-commerce is on the rise', *Marketing Charts*, 10 January 2020. Accessed 20 February 2022. www.marketingcharts.com/digital/social-media-111525

[28] Erica Gonzales, 'Kendall Jenner responds to her Fyre Festival involvement for the first time', *Haper's Bazaar*, 3 April 2019. Accessed 20 February 2022. www.harpersbazaar.com/celebrity/latest/a27028770/kendall-jenner-fyre-festival-responds/

Whilst influencers are supposed to make clear if they are being paid to advertise products in the UK, practically speaking, this is impossible to enforce. What's the difference between an influencer being paid in clothes to promote a brand, being 'gifted' clothes with no contract, buying them themselves in the hope of working with the brand, or just wearing them because they like the clothes, with zero expectation of money? Think of how many different scenarios there are every day like this on social media – *everything* you see on there is essentially an advertisement, even if it isn't officially 'sponsored'. If people aren't advertising a company, they're advertising themselves. Just think of how many people 'need it for work'.

Cybersecurity

As we can't trust what we see online, this makes us very vulnerable to people deliberately stealing money from us. This could range from hackers forwarding your emails to them and creating false payment pages, to having your social media account hacked and payments being made from your account. Just think of how many different websites your payment details are linked up to online. The devastating impact of this is how stupid and helpless it leaves us feeling, despite this being done by extremely intelligent professionals.

I recently had a shoot where 2 out of 3 women had been scammed that *week*. One received emails from what she thought was Facebook, giving her instructions on how to re-access her account and asking for ID, which she provided. She had direct debits set up from her bank account and child pornography posted on her page, blocking her from accessing her Facebook account. She couldn't figure out what was and wasn't Facebook, or any way to properly engage with them about the situation. We went through her accounts and changed all the passwords, switching on two-factor authentication, but it can be incredibly difficult to think straight if this happens.

The other woman had believed a video posted to her friends' Instagram account of him talking about a cryptocurrency investment scheme. She had a conversation with him over Instagram about it, and sent a payment to the scheme too. It was only when she was asked for her username and password that she realised there may be an issue, and fortunately called the person, who explained that he'd been hacked and had sent the testimonial video in the hopes of getting his money and details back. Instead, he was locked out of his account and the scammers were pretending to be him, but he was too embarrassed to tell anyone about it.

These situations show how easy it can be to fall into the traps of financial scams on social media, and how helpless it can leave you feeling. What we see online is not real, as in 'E is for Expectations', but we can easily forget this.

Earning money through social media

Social media and apps like Uber have resulted in a boom of self-employment, but this can be trickier than it looks on Instagram. Content creation can be extremely valuable to companies, but in a world where it seems like everybody is a creator, and we're lucky to get 'exposure' from brands in return for work, it can be very difficult to negotiate for yourself. Then it can be even more difficult to actually get the money you're owed for work, especially if this is from a company based in a different country to you!

Although working as an 'influencer' may look like a glamorous job of being well paid to promote products, the reality is probably as different as it is in modelling! Most models I know don't make enough money to survive financially, even those with good agents, because there is a huge oversupply of models in contrast to paying jobs. When I once accepted clothes from a brand in return for a social media shoot, I couldn't understand why my agent was so angry, but she explained that this had just set a new standard in lowering everybody's rates.

Friends of mine with hundreds of thousands of followers weren't charging to promote products, because they felt bad – despite the brands' websites they posted about crashing with demand as soon as they put up a post. They were working in shops and cafes, and part of what made them so popular online was that they weren't profiting from posting – they were authentic.

It's important to remember this if content creation is an industry you want to enter – you will have to sell yourself. Just like I struggled as a model with having to put my face to brands I didn't believe in (which I often wasn't told about in advance of the jobs being booked!), as a creator, you may have a similar lack of choice. You're selling your own values, and it can be very difficult to charge brands you believe in enough money to be able to survive financially. I'd really recommend checking out Stefanie Sword-Williams' book *'Fuck Being Humble'*, which has helped me significantly in becoming more confident in this area.

Whilst the virtual world offers us opportunities to make and spend money, the world's best engineers, marketing experts and behavioural psychologists are your competition, meaning that it's very likely to end up spending more than we intend to. The reality of starting a business can be very challenging, and involves much more than just setting up an Instagram account!

Tips

- Assess your finances. Can you dedicate an afternoon to writing down everything you've spent and earned in the last month across all bank accounts, in categories like 'subscriptions', 'groceries', 'entertainment', and so on? I do this on a weekly basis, and it's extremely empowering to know how much is going in and out of my accounts.
- Ensure you have two-factor authentication on all of your online accounts. This would require you to use a password

and another form of verification, such as your phone number or a code given by an authentication app.

- Assess your online accounts and passwords. You could use a secure platform to host these, ensuring every password is different and that you know what you do and don't have.
- If you're self-employed, I really recommend using 'QuickBooks' for managing your finances and creating invoices.
- Teach yourself about money from trusted sources, such as 'Your Juno' app, which focuses on financial empowerment education for women.
- Regularly review your subscriptions and delete any that you don't need or use. Don't wait to do it next time – do it now! Calculate how much these subscriptions add up to on a yearly basis.
- Create a budget for yourself by identifying your necessary basic spending, such as bills, and compare this to your monthly income.
- If you're in debt, consider talking to charities or organisations that can support you such as Debtors Anonymous.
- Avoid using habit forming apps such as 'Buy Now Pay Later' platforms, because these can hook you into long-term debt.
- Avoid any 'free' delivery or trial schemes. Having to pay even a little amount for something to be delivered can make us consider whether we *really* want something.
- Remove your payment card from your phone, or block certain websites from your internet browser, if you find that you're spending money subconsciously. Try to ask yourself whether you really want something before buying it.

- Write down things you want to buy in diary to buy 24 hours later. Designing a pause like this can be a good way of tricking our brains into thinking we've acted but allowing us to reflect later on potentially impulsive purchases.

- If you can, set up automatic payments to be deducted from your bank account to a savings account which is more difficult to access impulsively. If you're not sure, start small – even just £1 per week can make a significant difference over time.

- Avoid any online gambling websites, apps or 'quick win' investment schemes – remember, the house always wins.

- If you're sending a payment to someone online, especially someone you don't know, send £0.01 first and ask them to confirm receipt. It can be very easy for people to make a mistake in the bank details, and this simple act can save you a lot of stress down the line!

- Try to find a friend to go through your spending and earnings with each week, turning this into a routine. It's great to reflect on your successes, support each other with advice and to have the extra dose of accountability.

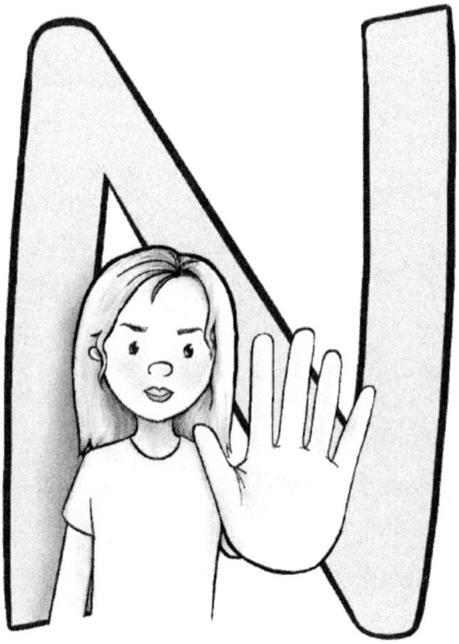

is for No

N is for No

Did you know?

- 1 in 5 teenagers who sent sexually explicit photographs of themselves because they were blackmailed or coerced into it, with 15% of surveyed 13-year-olds having experienced this behaviour.[29]

One of the best things about working in an office was the ability to leave my work there. Not taking my laptop home meant that I had evenings and weekends entirely free of obligations, where I was able to properly relax. In contrast, the Covid-19 lockdown meant that everybody started working from home. I'd wake up some days and turn my laptop on whilst still in bed, and carry on working until late in the evening. The lines between work and not work became very blurred, because I was theoretically able to work at all times – so why shouldn't I?

This is the world we're living in. We're accessible 24 hours a day by email and phone, so what excuse do we have for not replying to messages quickly enough? How do we set boundaries on the internet, when we're on zoom calls showing people into our homes? How do we separate out our work and relationships, fun and relaxation? Social media blends these concepts together into one, making it very hard to put ourselves first.

It can also give us the feeling of being watched at all times, as in 'O is for Objectification'. I once dated someone who wanted to speak on the phone every evening, who would then complain if he saw me

[29] ITV, 'One in five teenagers who sent 'sexts' pressured into it – survey' | ITV News, 19 June 2020. Accessed 17 March 2022.

appear online afterwards! This sense of constant surveillance can seep into all parts of our lives, such as feeling obligated to comment on certain friends' posts to ensure they don't get upset.

People pleasing

This is when we put others before ourselves and act out of 'feeling bad', or wanting to be 'nice'. Such behaviour generally comes with expectations, resulting in very unequal relationships. It can feel like subconsciously *choosing* to exploit yourself for others, in the hope that they'll like you.

The irony in this is that people rarely react the way we want them to, despite our best efforts – the only person's opinion we can control is ours. However, social media gives the illusion of being able to control this, in making our online interactions transactional. I was forever having to actively check my friends' profiles to make sure I hadn't missed one of their posts to comment on, which was made more annoying by the algorithm that most likely understood this and rarely showed their posts!

This kept a constant sense of guilt and unease in me that I'd missed an important update, or hadn't given them enough attention online in comparison to other people. In this way, people pleasing can keep us hooked on the apps, posting meaningless comments in the hope of receiving these back ourselves, as in 'V is for Validation'.

It can also make us exhausted, because we're spreading ourselves so thinly over so many people that we're unable to have actual relationships with anybody, as in 'F is for Friendships'. It is simply not possible to keep up to date with the lives or messages of hundreds of people, but social media can trick us into thinking we should be able to do this. As a result, we might say yes to too much, and have to back out later on, making us feel bad about ourselves.

People pleasing has become embedded into our society, which values 'busyness' and external displays of success over having time to relax away from screens, and being a 'good' person, employee, friend, family member and so on... essentially, being able to do it all. You are just a human being at the end of the day, and your first priority needs to be yourself.

The difficulty with lives so entrenched in social media is that we can become so used to seeing the needs of other people, that we forget about ourselves. It can be very easily to subconsciously replace our own needs and wants with theirs, subconsciously taking us away from who we are and how we want to be spending our life.

Avoiding exploitation online

If you're a creative, you'll recognise the frustration of being asked to do something for 'exposure'. After I was pressured to lose weight by an agency for 6 months and graduated to being able to go to castings, I learned that high fashion modelling, such as for magazines, doesn't pay anything at all. It was my 'privilege' to starve myself and work for free.

Social media drags us all into this world, where exposure has become an acceptable currency. I've seen people who aren't models be picked by huge brands to model for them and not be paid for it, because they're 'lucky' to get the photos! It confuses the lines between marketing ourselves and work we should be paid for, as in 'O is for Objectification'.

However, it's important to recognise this and the things that you don't want to do. This comes with identifying your own needs and values first, and then deciding what is aligned with what you want – not the other way around. Typically, whenever we do something that we are resenting in some way, we're likely to be ignoring a need of ours.

This is vital for situations where someone is making us feel uncomfortable, especially online. When I was growing up it was drummed into me to avoid speaking to people on the internet I didn't know in real life, but nowadays it's completely normal to connect with strangers all around the world every day, and potentially meet up with them. No matter how cool their profile might look, or how many photos or videos they post, it's vital to remember that *people are not always who they say they are*, as in 'M is for Money'.

When we're seeking approval from other people, we might present fake versions of ourselves back, and go against our own boundaries. As in 'X is for X-rated', this can lead us into situations we might regret in the future, such as sending explicit photos of ourselves.

Social media can make this seem like not such a big deal, because 'everyone does it'. It can make us feel like we're being unreasonable by not making quick, impulsive decisions and taking our time to think things through. Simply having tools like disappearing messages, such as on Snapchat, can make us feel like we're somehow being paranoid in not wanting to trust somebody on the internet. However, there's all sorts of ways that these tools can be manipulated, such as taking screen shots, and once something is on the internet, it's there forever.

Setting boundaries

When we set a boundary in a relationship, we're setting a standard of how we want to be treated. It's up to the other person to accept that if they want to continue being in a relationship with us. In the context of social media, this becomes much harder as we face a limitless number of interactions with other people throughout the day.

I used to feel so guilty for setting boundaries that I'd follow everyone back who followed me, swipe right for everyone on dating apps, accept any friend request, reply to any message, and help anyone who needed it. I lived a life I hated, because I completely ignored my own needs and 'felt bad' for everybody else except myself! I ended up dating and being friends with people I didn't even like, and prioritizing toxic people above those who genuinely cared about me, because those tended to be more understanding of my cancellations.

No is a complete sentence. It is not rude or offensive to not want to do something. It's not rude to reply to someone a few days later, or even to not reply at all, if you don't want to. This treats the delicate line with having basic respect for people, but once you respect yourself, you can treat others how you'd feel if they treated you. Would you be upset if a friend didn't reply to your text for 2 hours? Would you be upset if a person you didn't know didn't follow you back online?

Turning my Whatsapp notifications off changed my life dramatically, because I was no longer being distracted by people all of the time. I used to pride myself on replying instantly to every message, but now I *choose* when to even receive these messages, and live a life free of these distractions.

This can be important to recognise, because our avoidance to miss a single message or ever appear rude to anyone at all, can result in us being chained to our devices and apps. Friends of mine refused to delete Instagram from their phone in case they missed a message they needed to reply to. These hopes of new messages can often be an addiction in themselves, but they prevent us from taking control of our own time.

Boundaries are also important in deciding how much of ourselves we want to share online. Whilst we might share parts of our lives with our followers, such as what we're eating for breakfast, this doesn't mean we're under an obligation to post about our personal experiences. It can be difficult to draw the line between personal and professional content online, and in particular, to identify what we don't feel comfortable putting out to the world.

In general, it's advisable to avoid posting too much personal information online. This is especially important for security reasons, even if you're not mega famous. After I published *the Model Manifesto,* I had a man I didn't know message me on all different kinds of platforms asking to meet up. I blocked him, but he turned up to the launch events, where I'd fortunately blocked his name! Then he called my workplace and pretended to be calling about a work matter to get through reception, before he was put through to me and asked to come by my office!

Needless to say, this was terrifying and I went straight to the police. However, I was very fortunate that the situation didn't get worse. Social media can normalize things like posting pictures of our house, what we get up to in our free time, where we work, and how we spend our days, but this can leave us very dangerously exposed. It's important to remember that not everybody is entitled to connect with you, and you don't owe anybody any information!

You don't have to be friends with the whole world, and not everybody needs to like you. Something quite amazing happens when you start accepting this and protecting your energy – people respect you much more! Ultimately, having strong boundaries is a mark of respect to other people also, because we're communicating standards of how we expect ourselves to be treated, rather than expecting others to read our minds.

Social media places us all in the same pressure cooker of expectations, demands, and obligations, and to break free of it empowers other people to do the same.

<u>Tips</u>

- Assess your needs, wants and boundaries. What do you prioritize? For example, health, relationships, family, friends, and so on? How much of your life is in alignment to this?

- Imagine notifications or messages you receive on the internet as letters coming through your letter box – you'd very quickly be overwhelmed, especially if you had to reply to them all! The virtual world can distort our reality, but it doesn't mean it's something we should simply accept.

- What boundaries do you have in your relationships, and with the online world? Do you feel able to say no when you want to? How would these situations be ideally, if you didn't have to worry about anybody else?

- How can you take an action to uphold your boundaries? For example, deleting an app or sticking to a single time each day to check messages and reply, with an alarm after a certain period?

- When you need to communicate boundaries, it can helpful to say, 'when you do X, I feel Y. I would prefer it if you did Z.' This states what we are uncomfortable with and how we feel about it, without blaming the other person, and sets the standard for how we want to be treated.

- Do you know your limits? If someone refuses to respect your boundaries, can you change your behaviour accordingly, such as limiting your contact with them, depending on the context?

- Consider the language you use when communicating boundaries. For example, I have set the boundary of not replying to people straight away. I try to avoid apologising to them, because this automatically suggests that I've done something wrong, when in reality all I've done is avoid a distraction, allowing them to do the same!

- Remember that you owe your virtual audience nothing: these obligations are often very much in our head. On social media, I try to take time off without feeling bad for anyone, because I don't owe anyone my presence on there. By me taking a break, I allow other people to do the same.

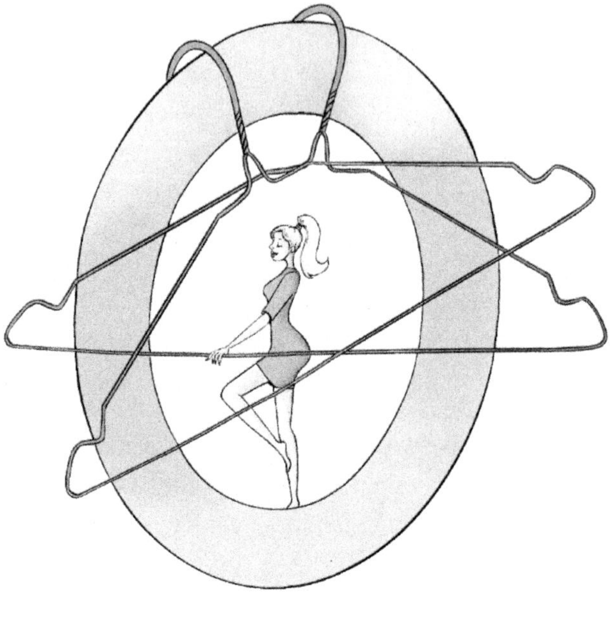

is for Objectification

O is for Objectification

Did you know?

- OnlyFans was found to be failing to prevent underage users from selling and appearing in explicit videos, with under-18s using fake identification to set up accounts. OnlyFans takes a 20% share of all payments in return for hosting the content that users pay to view.[30]

When I was a teenager, I was obsessed with being 'normal'. I collected data from people around me to understand how I could fit in and be liked. I studied the clothes I should wear, found out the 'cool' shops, learned how many times per week I should wash my hair, and the thoughts that I should and shouldn't say out loud. I had no idea who 'I' actually was until I hit my twenties and realised I'd lived my entire life for other people – constantly externalising and tweaking myself like a product.

Today, this concept of high school popularity has extended way past school and into our adult lives. Social media has made companies try to act like people, and people try to act like companies. It's so easy to let ourselves be dictated by the opinions of others – whether that's the amount of likes we get on Instagram, followers we have on TikTok, or unread emails waiting in our inbox. We can measure our worth as a human being according to how popular we believe ourselves to be – but this is never going to work.

For one, as in 'C is for Content', generally the most extreme content becomes the most popular – the algorithm doesn't measure by

---

[30] Chris Bell, Noel Titheradge, and Rianna Croxford, 'The children selling explicit videos on OnlyFans' - BBC News

standards of how symmetrical your haircut is, but how many people would have an emotional reaction to it, especially anger or fear. Also, many people have fake followings, as in 'I is for Influence'. It's a broken system to measure yourself by, even if it was possible to define what makes a human being 'better' than anyone else.

Branding

Even though we know these things, it can still be really difficult to be ourselves in a world where even the people we know in real life have got 'brand' versions of themselves online. What do you write in your bio on social media accounts? 'L is for Love' shows how difficult it is for us to portray mini versions of ourselves on single internet pages – presenting how we look in 3-5 photographs, and our interests, life aspirations, career, and everything else that's made up our entire existence on this planet in answers to a few curated questions.

The issue with branding yourself, is that you're objectifying yourself – you're seeing yourself as a product for an audience, rather than just being you. This is how I've treated myself as a model since the age of 13, where people regularly spoke about me as though I wasn't in the room, as though my body parts were objects, like pieces of furniture. They'd pore over the number of split ends I had, the exact symmetry of my eyebrows (I once spent 3 hours having these re-shaped by a make-up artist who'd painted them black on a shoot – the problem was obviously theirs, but it still left me thinking I had uneven eyebrows!), and the whiteness of my eyes.

I once had a wedding dress shoot where I was called too thin, too fat, too tall, too small, too unsymmetrical, too flat chested, and too curvy, all in one day. This is because the team were looking at how the dresses fit me, rather than thinking about my feelings. When you're a model, your body is essentially available to be rented out for the day to the highest bidder. Your feelings don't matter. You don't get a say in whether you hate your hair and make up, or whether you'd rather not wear a degrading outfit, or do a degrading pose. As in 'N is for No', if you do, your entire livelihood is at risk.

It literally feel like being a human Barbie doll. I developed extreme disassociation from my body, where I can easily stand in a room of 20 people who are insulting me and tune out of what they're saying. As in 'D is for Disordered Eating', model agencies often tell you how you should change your entire appearance after scouting you, which is something many people often accept without question.

It's only been on the odd occasions when stylists asked if it was okay to touch me before shoving their hands down my trousers to readjust the line of my underwear, that I realised maybe this wasn't normal behaviour. It filters out to the rest of your life – I had no boundaries with anyone, and offered myself up as a product to be used in the same way in my personal relationships. We all have feelings, and even though I was able to switch them off for days at a time, they still existed, launching me into a deep depression and making it incredibly difficult for me to live my own life, because I was so used to other people's opinions rather than my own.

This disassociation also translated to social media. Models suddenly needed to be more than a blank canvas, but to have a personality, showcased online to our plentiful followers. I'd post pictures of me from years ago modelling, posting them with a caption to wish everyone a 'Happy Monday', just to make it look like I was busy. I became an active participant in objectifying myself, rather than mentally stepping outside of the room.

Whenever I saw my own modelling photos, I would rip them apart, criticising myself like I was an art critique inspecting a painting, seeking out imperfections before debating whether to post it on my profile. A friend saw me do this once and became very upset at how horrible I was about myself, but it didn't even feel like me in the photos. I didn't feel any emotional connection to them other than the ability to find all the negatives, which I'd never have done to anyone else's photo!

Social media can allow us to objectify our entire lives, not just how we look. An agent once told me how they monitored their models' social media accounts as otherwise they'd post pictures of themselves eating pizza and clients would call up to complain. When every single aspect of your life becomes a brand and who you are in real life stops being acceptable, we lose ourselves. As in 'F is for Friendships', this can also impact our relationships with other people in real life, turning everything into a transaction.

This is the reality we ALL live in now, whether you're a professional model or not. Almost everyone I know has a 'brand', the types of photos they post, a tone of voice they use online – even if they don't realise it themselves. Every time we post something online about us or our lives, we're looking for a reaction, and objectifying ourselves in the process – opening ourselves up to external validation. We're all put in the position of evaluating our own posts, and trying to figure out how we could do 'better'. When we live like this subconsciously and automatically, it can lead to disassociating from ourselves in exactly the same way as I did as a model – we stop being us, and start being a bystander, who's often pretty mean!

This is the danger of becoming an 'influencer' – the ability to become 'famous' depends on your ability to disconnect from yourself and your life, to sell a curated version of yourself that is decided by other people. You become a brand, not a person.

Living for an audience

When I graduated from University, I didn't know what to 'do' with my life. So I just followed what my social media feed showed me, and ended up in Australia, as in 'I is for Influence'. Once I'd got there, I became incredibly depressed. It felt like there were different versions of me – the one that would go and buy papayas to photograph them on the beach, thinking out captions and potential photos to post online, and the other, who was judging myself. I hated myself for presenting this life on the internet to people I hardly even knew, trying to get validation from them. I become as one-dimensional as my photographs and didn't know how to experience life outside of that world.

I ended up feeling suicidal, but once I deleted my Instagram account, I felt better, as in 'Q is for Quitting'. This is because I didn't want to live in this way anymore, not because I didn't want to live at all. Once I'd lost my imaginary audience I was able to live my life for myself, even with my senses coming back, such as noticing smells and sounds that I didn't notice before. I de-objectified myself.

However, this can happen automatically without us even realising. I used to go to dance classes where the entire point of them was to record a video of yourself at the end to post online. Everybody came in incredible outfits and a full face of make-up. This wasn't fun – it was work. I saw how people linked their self-worth to the number of likes they got on these videos, which takes the entire point out of doing an 'empowering' dance class! In contrast, I used to go to dance classes in pitch black darkness, which were one of my favourite ever activities, because no one could see me doing my most 'interesting' moves.

Despite these classes being dark, I noticed my mind starting to obsess over how I could post about it. I realised I had a literal Instagram filter in my brain, that jumped out to capture fun moments and tried to objectify them. I went off Instagram again for a few months, re-entering into my own life, but always noticed how it was the 'fun' experiences, like a holiday or hanging out with friends, that I wanted to post online. We can easily objectify our entire lives in this way, when we're living for the posts, rather than the experiences.

When we objectify ourselves, we can easily find ourselves lost, numb and depressed, as we stop being able to enjoy life. If we're constantly looking for reasons outside of ourselves to post online, then we'll be on an endless treadmill, forgetting that no one is going to look after us but *us*. The difference between brands and people, is that brands don't have any feelings. They don't mind 'selling out', because they've got changeable business values and goals, whereas human beings have morality and a soul. Our personalities and messy human emotions are impossible to stuff into a box to be neatly sold to an audience.

When you are what you do

Have you ever noticed that one of the first questions new people will ask you is what you 'do'? How do we separate ourselves from jobs when we *are* the job? For example, I often felt too embarrassed to tell people that I was modelling, because I assumed they thought I was arrogant in some way, or lying. The automatic reaction of people is often to require proof – asking when I last worked, or which clients I worked for, or which agency I was with. They'd nearly always ask me what I'm going to do 'after' modelling, or what else I 'do'. It was a great contrast to say I worked in law, because no one cared!

Many creatives have had similar experiences, of following their passions but not being sure how to commercialize and 'brand' this. A very talented photographer once told me he wasn't able to continue, because he'd been shooting 'influencers' in an attempt to build his portfolio and book more work, but hated contributing to this lifestyle.

Social media measures our 'success' in our jobs by how good we are at marketing ourselves, creating content, and understanding algorithms, not by our real talents. This can unfortunately leave many brilliantly talented people feeling bad about their ability to do their job well because of how much engagement they get online – there is no correlation!

Speaking to teenagers, I see how difficult it is for them in this world, where they're expected to have a fresh stream of content – but most of what they 'do' is go to school. They're not being photographed in magazines or able to book flights to take photos on a beach. They're just trying to figure out who they are and what they want to do in life, and social media shows them an endless stream of 'perfect' careers as influencers, placing impossible pressures on them, as in 'E is for Expectations'.

The reality is that we all change throughout our lives. Most of us will have several different careers, and when we try to objectify ourselves through social media in marketing ourselves, this can feel very conflicting. When we build up a following around one certain aspect of our lives, it can feel very difficult to change our 'brand', as in 'N is for No'. I felt this myself in returning to modelling after writing the Model Manifesto, despite now modelling in line with the principles I set out in the book – social media distorts these complex realities into bitesize content.

This isn't limited to creative jobs, as 'professional' platforms like LinkedIn are becoming more popular in posting personal updates about our work and achievements in return for likes and shares, with the added opportunity of potentially attracting new work. When we link what we 'do' so closely with who we 'are', it can feel very challenging to separate them – but these are very different things.

For example, when I wrote a book about ADHD and later read an article about Autism that resonated very strongly with me, I freaked out and thought I'd somehow been lying to people without even realising, questioning my entire diagnosis. Fortunately, these days I'm able to simply step back from the internet, as in 'Q is for Quitting', and take a more balanced approach.

Having now had well over 15 different Instagram accounts, I know that we can start over as many times as we want – nobody ultimately cares for very long, but we can just trick ourselves into imagining that they do.

Online marketing is important, but you should be in control of it – not the other way around. Remember that these platforms give us an entirely false sense of success – we can objectify ourselves to be as famous as we want, but if we're not enjoying the life we're posting online, what's the point?

Tips

- Assess how you feel about yourself as a 'brand'. What do you 'do', and who are you? How do you portray yourself online, and how do you feel about yourself in reality? Do you feel like these versions of yourself match up?
- Consider how you feel if content you post online doesn't get as much feedback as you'd hoped. How about if it went viral? How much of your life would you say is being lived for you, versus an imaginary audience?
- If you post about your work online, how can you create boundaries between your personal and professional self? I'd very strongly advise having two separate accounts for this, if possible.
- How can you remove yourself from the feedback on your posts, to share what you want to in a way that feels aligned with your values, without being dependent on validation? For example, if you have a business online, can you plan out your content using an automatic calendar to schedule and post content?
- Try out new experiences relating to what you enjoy doing, and be present in them, instead of thinking about them from the outside. Things like yoga and meditation can be great for this.
- Identify what your reasons and hopes are when posting content online. The difference between creative expression and self-objectification can easily become blurred on social media!

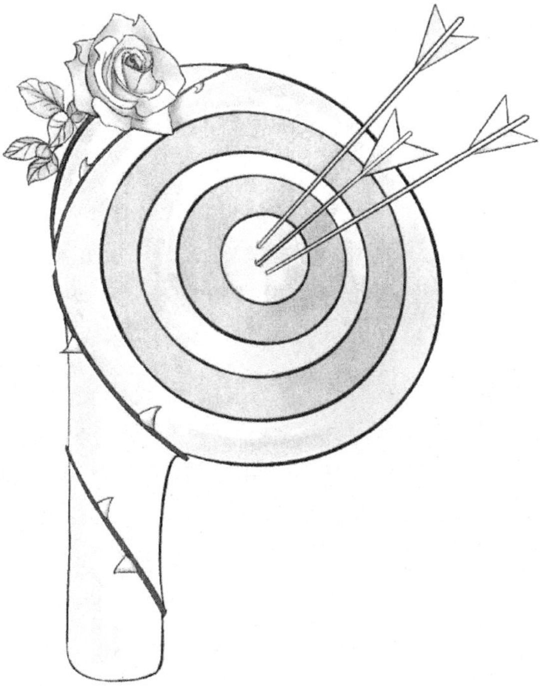

is for Perfectionism

P is for Perfectionism

- A study found perfectionism is a vulnerability factor for things such as depression and poor body image in female adolescents following appearance-focused social comparison when using social media.[31]

Above anything else, social media presents to us the lie of perfection. Seeing highlights reels of people's lives leads us to believe that happiness can be achieved, if we only looked a certain way, achieved a certain number of followers, or had a certain lifestyle. From 'perfect' bodies to friendships, nights out to holidays, what we see on social media is not real. Just think of how many completely, 100% perfect experiences you've had in real life!

For example, we could look back on a photograph of us at a festival and remember only how brilliant the music was, and how happy we were dancing with our friends. We've forgotten the hours spent queuing for food and the toilets or getting lost and our phone running out of battery, leading to us having a panic attack. In real life, these challenges are what make our experiences so enjoyable, because we've overcome them, as in 'R is for Resilience', but it's easy to forget how horrible they were at the time.

This can lead us to not only comparing ourselves to other people's lives, but also our own past experiences. For example, we can look back on the posts of us in a previous relationship and be fooled into

---

[31] Marianne Etherson, thomas Curran, Martin Smith, Simon Sherry, Andrew Hill, 'Perfectionism as a vulnerability following appearance-focussed social comparison: A multi-wave study with female adolescents' - ScienceDirect, February 2022. Accessed 17 March 2022: https://www.sciencedirect.com/science/article/pii/S0191886921007340

only remembering the good times, beating ourselves up, but we've forgotten the reasons that this person is no longer in our lives. This can leave us in an impossible and endless state of trying to control our lives to be 'perfect', like what we see on social media – despite this not existing in the first place. We must consciously and regularly remind ourselves of reality, otherwise we can work towards completely fake standards.

Although we've got far more opportunities than our grandparents did, from finding a potential soulmate anywhere in the world, as in 'L is for Love', to becoming famous overnight by going on a reality television show, as in 'I is for Influence', or changing our faces, as in 'S is for Surgery', these don't necessarily make us any happier. Instead, they can make us overwhelmed with limitless versions of 'perfection'. How can we achieve the perfect life we see on social media if we can always have something else to aim for?

Happily ever after

Have you ever had the experience of being extremely hungry at a restaurant, whilst waiting for your food to come? The highs and lows of watching other people's food come out before yours can feel like an emotional rollercoaster. When yours does finally come, you feel the elated burst of happiness and excitement, your mouth literally salivating.

After the first bite of magical food, that feeling wears off. We forget how hungry we were. Maybe the food isn't even as good as we expected it to be. We check our phones and stop really tasting or thinking about the food we're eating. We start thinking about what to eat for dessert.

When we get new things, from a new phone, to new clothes, to lip filler, we adjust very quickly, and these things become normal. This about the worst thing we can be in the days of social media and influencing, so we seek to make our lives 'perfect'. After I graduated from university, I spent years trying to perfect myself and my life, to find the 'perfect' career, thinking this would make me happy.

All it did was make me horribly depressed. Everything in life has good and bad parts of it, and if we're unable to accept the bad parts in pursuit of something perfect, we end up having nothing. Even when we think we've found something perfect, this always wears off.

This is because of evolution and dopamine – it helps us to keep seeking out new experiences and growing. If we suddenly achieved our dreams tomorrow, what would we do then? If we were completely satisfied after eating a delicious meal out and never became hungry again, then we'd never eat again, and wouldn't survive very long!

However, social media tricks us into forgetting this, and believing that perfection is within our reach, which will grant us the magical wish of being 'happy'. Posting our 'normal' lives online won't get as much attention as posts about our extreme experiences, so we can often be presented with a world of alternative options that might make us feel happier, every time we look at our phones. I remember sitting on a beach in Thailand scrolling through my phone wishing I'd actually gone on holiday to Cambodia or Bali!

Just as we don't all like the same type of fruit, we don't all have the same standards of perfection. This is crucially important to remember if you're on this treadmill – what might be 'perfect' to you, won't necessarily make you any happier.

When I became extremely unwell and lost all the weight I had been previously pressured to lose for modelling, finally reaching the 'target goal' I'd been trying to reach for the previous 10 years, my family literally burst into tears upon seeing me because they thought I was going to die. My skin went grey, my bones stuck out of me, and I covered up with huge t-shirts.

I'd reached the 'target' measurements that I'd been given by the modelling industry as perfection for over 10 years, and never looked worse. However, on a catwalk or during a professional photograph, clothes would hang off my frail body like they were hanging on a coat hanger, exactly as they were designed on paper. The other parts of my body, like my face and hair, could be styled by top professionals or photoshopped beyond recognition. This is virtually impossible for anyone to achieve or maintain, which is why it's held up as 'perfection'.

Capitalism

This is the 'hedonistic treadmill', where we get one thing and need another. It doesn't have an end in sight, but running on it makes us feel like we have a tiny bit of control over our happiness – that if we just had a new outfit, or a new house, or a new nose, we'd be happier. When we get the hit of reality and reminder that we're still not happy, even with the car we've just spent a year's salary on, it's not a sign that something is seriously wrong with us, but a sign that we are human beings.

In school, I pushed myself incredibly hard to get good marks, because I had to be perfect. I didn't study subjects I enjoyed, I only did ones that 'looked good' for university. Then I studied law, because it seemed like the 'best' option to do. I thought these things would make me perfect, but they just made me feel like an imposter, because I didn't really understand what I was studying – I'd just figured out how to do well in exams.

I also felt terrified of getting older, even as a teenager. I'd started modelling age 13, but I met another girl who'd been scouted at 11 by a top London agency and told to come in for weekly measurements, to try and hold off puberty. As a 14-year-old, they said she was too fat to model.[32] As in 'D is for Disordered Eating', society holds these

[32] This model has now set up a brilliant company called Period Parcels to empower girls getting their periods: www.periodsparcels.com

child versions of ourselves as the standard of perfection, because they are unachievable. As in 'B is for Beauty', capitalism thrives from making us feel like we have a problem that needs fixing.

This is even worse in today's world, where we're literally comparing ourselves to dimensions that don't exist. For example, some fashion brands have started to use virtual fashion models, made using artificial intelligence! As a teenager, I'd already started spending hours looking in the mirror worrying about potential wrinkles and tensing my stomach all of the time to try and grow abs. When someone mentioned my 'wrinkles' to me at my graduation dinner, I felt the impending doom of being a less-than-perfect woman descend on me, of being old. Keeping up with the standards of perfection that don't exist in the first place leave us feeling miserable in our real-life existence, as in 'E is for Expectations'.

Control

Trying to control things that can't be controlled, like the way we look, is a slippery path. It's how we end up with eating disorders and self-harming, as an outlet for the lack of control we feel in our day to day lives. Feeling like at least we can control the harm we do to ourselves can lead to a momentary feeling of shame, realness and perfection rolled into one, as in 'O is for Objectification'.

These methods of fake control will have lasting effects on you for your entire life, just like getting tattoos or plastic surgery. There is no ultimate perfection to be found when you look or feel a certain way. Even the most beautiful woman in the world will have times when she feels ugly - probably more often than you can imagine. You can't erase the pores from your skin, or your organs from your body. Even if you could look like Kim Kardashian as she appears on her Instagram, you still wouldn't be happy all the time.

Life happens to us, and we can't control it. Once we solve one problem, a different one pops up in its place. No one in the world is 100% happy, which is a good thing – this is what keeps us developing as people, and having all of the different experiences that make us human.

Imposter syndrome

Part of the problem with the perfect lives that we see on social media, is that it can make us feel like if we can't do something perfectly, it's not worth doing it all. If we can't be famous singers, there's no point in singing, if we're rejected by model agencies, we aren't 'models', if we can't be an award-winning actor, there's no point acting. As children we do these things for fun, and as we get older, they somehow get ripped away from us by a world that focuses on what we can do as 'work'.

I've written books about my personal experiences in life, because this is how I've processed and understood them for myself. I'm not a supermodel, model agency owner, psychiatrist, psychologist, behavioural scientist, tech guru, social media expert, or anything else – I'm just someone who's figured out ways to overcome some of the things I write about, sometimes. I've experienced the highs and lows of the worlds I write about, deep dived into research on how to fix myself, and written it out to process it.

Sharing these experiences with the rest of the world is an afterthought, to help others who might be going through the same thing, or further behind this path than me, thinking that if they achieve certain things like being famous on the internet it will make them happy. The positive feedback I've had about my books make me very happy I've shared my ramblings with the world, but I also get bouts of severe imposter syndrome, such as immediately after publishing *ADHD: an A to Z,* and misspelling ADHD!

I was so embarrassed that I tried to figure out how to unpublish the book – which went on to be the foundation of my career as an ADHD Coach! Feeling like we need to do another course or get an external stamp of approval holds us back from being able to do what we want to do, but having gotten a law degree, I can confirm that this doesn't make you feel any less of an Imposter. What I've learned is that everybody feels like an imposter, no matter how long they've been in their job, or how many letters they have after their name. We're all simply making it up as we go along.

Nowadays, I try to embrace this feeling of being an imposter, and ask as many questions as I can. Having successfully done a job in mental health and immigration law for 2 years during the pandemic, knowing absolutely zero about these areas before I started, I now trust myself to be able to understand how to work out to do most things, as in 'R is for Resilience'.

Today, perfection for me is feeling happy with my decisions, and accepting my life for how it is. Nothing will ever be truly 'done' – I know that if I ever finish editing this book and publish it, new work will start of having to promote it. I could literally continue writing and promoting it forever, holding myself to the standard of needing to write a fourth book. Our brains are constantly making up thoughts, but when we realise that we have a part in choosing which ones to believe, everything changes. I can give myself the deadline of tomorrow to finish this book, or it can be next year – it's completely up to me, just as your life is completely up to you.

By knowing that nothing will ever be truly 'done', we can allow ourselves to live life at our own pace. This isn't the same as settling for situations that make us feel mostly unhappy, but searching for a life that feels happy in the small moments, because these are what make up the rest of our lives.

Questioning our beliefs, decisions and inner dialogue, can help us remind ourselves over and over again: perfection does not exist. Accepting ourselves as we are, and our lives, is a path to much more fulfilling happiness than the ladder of perfection. It's easy to trick ourselves into believing we've got forever, but our time on this earth is very short (approximately 4000 weeks!), and we might as well enjoy it rather than beating ourselves up.

We're all here on this world with no roadmap, and no one's going to hold us to a life checklist when we die. The point of life is to live it, as imperfectly as possible, because this is how we learn and grow!

Tips

- Assess your standards of perfectionism. How much of your life do you live just for 'fun'? How often do you feel like you should be being productive? What does this mean to you?

- What does perfection mean to you? If you achieved the things you wanted, then what would you do? How would your life be different?

- How can you notice if you're holding yourself to an impossible standard of perfectionism? For example, do you have certain thoughts, procrastinate, or overwork yourself? What actions can you take to slow down and remind yourself that perfection doesn't exist, and done is better than perfect?

- Can you set yourself a new standard of 'perfect', to be simply listening to what you need in each moment, and following that?

- Try out mindfulness and meditation. As perfectionism is an addiction to trying to control something that doesn't exist, focus on the only thing you can control in life: how you choose to respond to it.

- Identify something to try that you're not already good at. When we're happy to be bad at something, we can do anything, as in 'R is for Resilience'.

- Can you break an overwhelming task down into chunks? For example, rather than feeling like you need to do everything right now, how can you break it down into trying something out, with no obligations?

- If you feel paralysed by different ideas, simply write them down in a notebook and pick one to focus on at a time. You don't necessarily need to finish writing your book for it to be done – it's just about following what interests us each day.

- Try journaling every day and writing about what you feel grateful for. You could also write a 'done' list of everything you've done that day, which always seems much more than I realise! Just because we *can* do a lot, doesn't meant that we should. How can you prioritize rest and breaks?

- Keep a list of your successes and moments of happiness in life, and reflect back on it when you're feeling negatively about yourself. How can you focus on how far you've come, instead of how far you have to go?

- Remind yourself that you're perfect exactly as you are. Do the things you want to do today, and don't worry about how good or bad they are – just do them for the experience of doing them, and enjoy your life. You don't need to change or fix yourself, prove anything to the world, or yourself. Please don't put your self-worth in the hands of something that doesn't even exist.

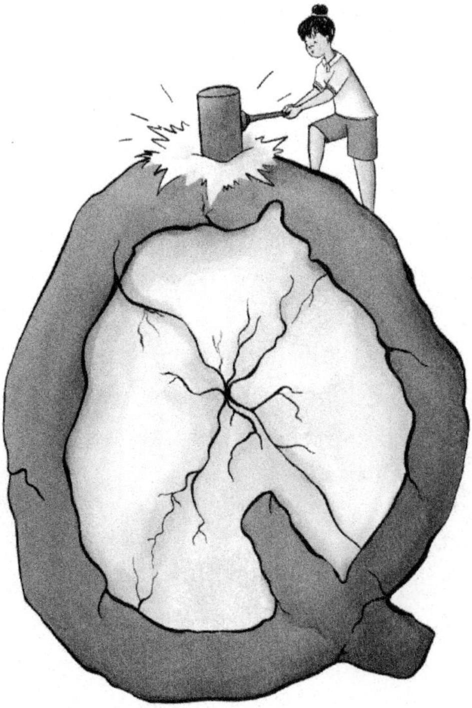

is for Quitting

Q is for Quitting

Did you know?

- Researchers found that deactivating Facebook can result in more in-person time with friends and family, an increase in one's daily moods and life satisfaction, and for the average user, an extra hour per day of relaxation. [33]

The first time I deleted my Instagram account, I felt free. Gone was the ability to check my notifications, the real and fake followers, the anxiety about what to post, the constant comparisons with other people. I wrote a blog post about it, not expecting anyone to read it, which went viral. Then I became a bit addicted to blogging, trying to get the same high. A few months later, I was back on Instagram.

Quitting anything, especially an addiction, is difficult to sustain if your environment doesn't change. It took me a long time to quit binge drinking and smoking, but this ultimately came from no longer putting myself in situations where everybody was doing the same. If I'd tried quitting whilst still going clubbing 3 times a week, I wouldn't have lasted very long! It's also easy for new unhealthy habits to pop up instead of our original habits that give us similar dopamine hits, such as different platforms.

There are a lot of positives to social media, not least the ability to connect with a huge number of people all over the world. Our options shouldn't be to quit the internet completely or be fully

---

[33] Hunt Allcott, Luca Braghieri, Sarah Eichmeyer and Matthew Gentzkow, 'The Welfare Effects of Social Media', November 8 2019, Stanford University. Accessed 17 March 2022: www.web.stanford.edu/~gentzkow/research/facebook.pdf

addicted – there should be a middle ground. Personally, I try to take a break when I notice I'm using it in unhealthy ways, and use social media in a conscious, purposeful way, instead of letting it use me.

Deleting your accounts

Can you imagine what would happen if your favourite social media platform disappeared overnight? Whilst we place a huge amount of emphasis on social media, the truth is that there's always other options. We might need to 'start again' on them, but ultimately, the platforms that feel like our entire worlds today might not even exist in 5 years. As in 'R is for Resilience', this is important to remember not to link our self-worth too closely to one platform.

When I deleted my Instagram, I assumed that was the end of my career as a model, but I'd hit breaking point. I was surprised to find that nobody cared as much as I thought they would, I carried on booking modelling work completely fine, and I didn't miss anything. When you don't know what's happening on social media, you don't care. I also felt different physically, noticing beauty in things I hadn't seen previously, like the sun shining through clouds, and noticed my sense of smell strengthening, as in 'Z is for Zen'.

I was a much happier person without Instagram, with a lot more time and head space. I hung out with friends and met new people without knowing or caring how many followers they had, did jobs without feeling the need to document it, and lived my life for me. Not having an account meant I felt much less insecurity or competition with other people, because I wasn't playing the game.

When I deleted my Facebook account, my relationships with my family and friends improved dramatically. I stopped having arguments with them about their opinions I disagreed with or getting frustrated by what I thought were provocative posts, because I couldn't see them. It's very easy to infer meaning onto the statuses we see of people we already know in real life, and to take everything we see personally, when often these things might not even be about us.

I lost touch with people that I'd never really been friends with anyway, such as people I went to school with, but I became much closer with the ones who mattered. As in 'F is for Friendships', I realised I'd somehow prioritised keeping up with my collective 'audience' rather than the people I knew in real life. Not having an account forced us all to make a bit more effort, which is really what relationships are: commitment. For social events, I have to be actively invited, rather than added to an event page I'd inevitably click 'attending' and forget about, double booking plans by the time the day arrived. The people whose events I'd want to go to always invite me – if they don't, then I don't know about it!

I'm very glad I deleted both of my Facebook and Instagram accounts, because these wiped a slate clean for me. Deleting your accounts proves to you that you have a life outside of social media, and the earth keeps spinning even if your accounts get deleted. You carry on earning a living, having connections with other people, and living your life – you just get bombarded with less information about people you might not care about so much, and aren't held to a past version of yourself that might no longer reflect who you are today.

This is a great option if you're feeling heavily reliant on your online persona and want to start afresh. If nothing else, it's a great way to reset your social media use and live a 'worst case scenario' of a life without the validation that may be tied to your virtual world, leaving you as nothing more than a normal human being. Ironically, I've found this has made me more interesting to people because they feel more relaxed around me, without the need to worry about our dual relationship on social media. You can always make new accounts in the future, as I have, many times!

Deactivating your accounts

Deactivating your accounts means they're not completely deleted forever, with all content gone, but your account is taken offline temporarily. If you reactivate it, everyone you follow may be notified that you've returned, which stops me from spontaneously deactivating and reactivating it every day. There's also something about mentally deactivating the account that stops me from spontaneously going back on.

Deactivating your accounts can be a really good tool to do that isn't so extreme as deleting them, but just enabling you to take a break and refresh your mind with reality for a while. If you have something you want to do but are struggling with being distracted, just try deactivating your most addictive social media accounts and see what happens. By setting yourself different limits each time, such as a day, week, or month, you can test your own resilience and compare the difference in how you feel.

Ask someone else to change your password

I used to do this as a teenager when I needed to study for my exams. I'd ask someone I trusted to change my Facebook password and post a status to say I was staying off to study for my exams, as I knew how much harder I needed to work having been unable to concentrate in classes all year. This combination was very effective, as I had nothing else to do but study!

This might work for you if you want a break but don't want your profile to disappear, such as if you run a business account. You could schedule posts and ask someone else to oversee this.

Delete your apps / turn off your notifications

Social media apps have been designed to be used on your phone, as features such as endless scrolling and bubble notifications make using them in this way much more addictive and enjoyable than an internet browser. Our brains can also move so quickly when we open our phones that it can be like entering a maze without even realising, as hours later we find ourselves scrolling on apps we don't even remember opening!

This is easily solved by deleting the apps from your phone, or hiding them, so you have to consciously type them in to search. You can also disable notifications, which is a great way of giving you control over deciding how you want to use your phone, rather than having it decided for you. I'd strongly advise deleting any apps from your homepage which make you feel bad about yourself, such as ones that edit your photos or tell you who's unfollowed you!

If the thought of this makes you feel uncomfortable, this is a good sign that you should probably give it a go! It's easy for apps to become self-soothing in a way, as our 'go to' activities whenever we're feeling slightly uncomfortable, but this is the problem: we need to be conscious when we're using them, because our entire self-esteem is at stake. Going on TikTok is not the same as watching a movie – we don't know what we're going to see, or how it's going to affect us. What we see is being continuously tweaked to be as addictive as possible, and it takes an invisible wrestling match to get off.

By committing to using the apps on desktop browsers only, you can still check in with the platforms, but without being manipulated by these addictive tools as featured on your phone.

Block websites from your phone

The only challenge with getting off apps, is noticing what pops up instead. When our brains are used to a certain level of dopamine hits in response to subconsciously seeking these out, it can look elsewhere without us even necessarily realising.

Whenever I deactivate my social media accounts, I find myself desperately seeking out stimulation from online shopping or news.

It’s like my brain wants to see something new, and is craving the hit of anticipation and excitement.

It’s good to pre-emptively stop this from happening by blocking websites that you might spend too much of your valuable time on in advance. This includes social media websites, as the temptation to download the app and delete it again when we’re on our phones might be too much to resist!

You can also use a program called ‘Freedom’ to block access to certain websites and apps across your phone and laptop for specified periods of time, which I strongly recommend. Failing this, you can use a physical ‘phone safe’ like I do!

Mute, unfollow, unfriend, and block people who make you feel bad

We all have our own insecurities, and most likely, someone in the world looks at your social media profile to compare themselves to you, just as we do to others. Whilst we can compare ourselves to the fantasy lives of celebrities, the people we know in real life can often be a much more triggering source of negative comparisons and feelings, as in ‘J is for Jealousy’.

Whilst we can draw a line between a world-famous celebrity and us, it’s harder to do so with the people we know, because this seems more achievable. This can easily spiral into unhealthy obsessions that leave us feeling guilty and confused. I had most of my friends muted on my social media accounts, because I just didn’t want to feel this odd sense of competition with them, as in ‘F is for Friendships’.

It's good to block people who won’t realise you’ve blocked them (such as famous people), as it’s so easy to subconsciously find ourselves on their accounts when we’re feeling bad. Unfollowing and unfriending people as the next level down – people who on the balance of probabilities, won’t realise or care, and muting everybody who makes you feel even slightly insecure about yourself. As in ‘N is for No', you are not obligated to anybody to keep up to date with their online posts.

If you're worried about people that you know realising, you could just say you're trialling a break from viewing stories / other people's posts / social media all together. The measure of a good friend is not someone who is up to date with our Instagram feed – it's someone who's there for us when we need them, and who supports us in real life.

Outsource

If you can, delegate your social media management. Programs such as Canva can automatically upload your posts on certain days, which worked really well for me for a while. However, it was always when I logged on to view the engagement that it became addictive again. I lost several weekends of my life making and planning my social media content, which I often ignored and posted spontaneously anyway, as in 'P is for Perfectionism'!

However, this can work really well if you have more restraint than me. If you can set a time each day to schedule your posts and go on to check messages, with a degree of separation from how 'well' they're doing, this can be a very healthy way to engage with social media. Another option I've tried is hiring a social media manager / personal assistant to upload pictures for me, but embarrassingly, it ended up pretty similarly as I just did it all myself anyway!

Some people find social media more problematic than others. For example, I know that I have to resort to extreme measures like writing this book because I can't control it, which might be something to do with my dopamine-hunting ADHD brain. Others might enjoy social media but find it annoying that they sometimes end up comparing themselves to others without realising. Ultimately, it's all about figuring out what works for you, and what kind of life you want to live, utilising the benefits whilst consciously being aware of your exposure to the negatives.

Take one small step today that will help you make the changes you want to see, and repeat. If you fall off the wagon, get back on it! You're literally working against teams of the world's top experts in keeping you hooked, but ultimately, you're in control of your own choices.

Tips

- Do a self-assessment: how much time do you spend on screens each day? How do you feel about this?
- How long could you go without going on your favourite social media platform? Can you challenge yourself to take a tiny step to be more conscious in how you use it, such as doing something else before opening the profiles in the morning?
- Try tracking your screen-time across all screen times for a week, and multiply it by 52. How would you feel if someone told you you'd lose this many hours from the next year?
- What would you do with your life if you had these hours back? What would you change if you could?
- Create a bucket list of experiences you want to have in life. It can be anything from going to a certain country or trying out a new activity. Can you make an effort to try and do one of these within the next month?
- Take pre-emptive action that will help you stick to your goals in using social media more consciously, such as adapting your environment accordingly, such as keeping your phone away from your desk when you want to focus, or charging it outside of your bedroom at night.
- Try out a 'screen detox' one day per week, such as on the weekend. You could give your screens to somebody else for the day and go on an adventure!

- Try one of the methods listed in this chapter, such as deleting apps from your home screen, for a certain number of days in the week. Figure out what works for you – it's your life.

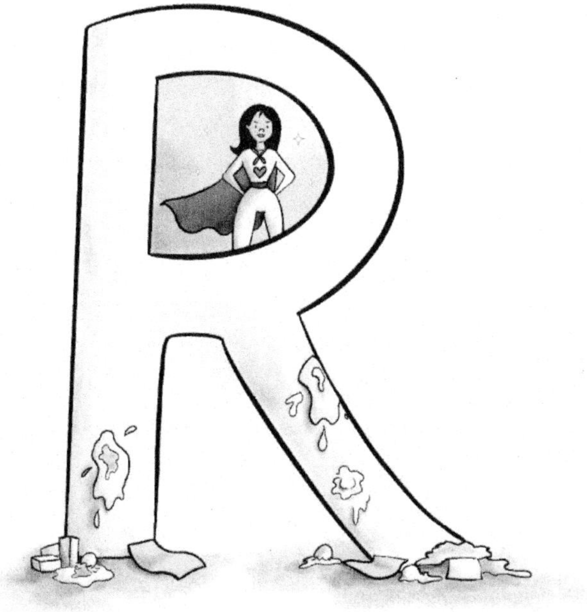

is for Resilience

R is for Resilience

Did you know?

- Children have a much harder time reacting to bad emotions. We usually adapt as adults into being resilient, but this is harder for younger generations, as they're exposed to constant negative interactions on social media. 47% of 12-to-19-year-olds got their social, professional, sexual and physical goals from Instagram, and that negative wellbeing sets in the moment they don't feel they measure up.[34]

Many people I talk to don't do what they really want to do in life in case they fail. Others don't share their opinions with others out of fear of getting it wrong, whilst some have pinned their entire self-worth on achieving certain arbitrary goals outside of their control. For many, the things they want to do aren't 'acceptable' in the frameworks they're currently living in, so these seem impossible.

When I left my law job last year to become an ADHD coach, other people in my life thought I was making a terrible decision, as this definitely wasn't the 'done' thing. However, I knew that I'd survived 5 years of being self-employed before, and even though I'd worried constantly about not making enough money to pay my rent each month, I always did. Having survived before meant that I knew I could survive again. Within a few weeks, I was thriving, much to the amazement of everyone else!

---

[34] Marie-Claire Chappet, 'Have we been brain-jacked by Instagram? As we're given the option to hide likes, we investigate how the 'gram has rewired our brains for good...', Glamour Magazine, 26 May 2021. Accessed 17 March 2022: www.glamourmagazine.co.uk/article/instagram-effect-on-brain, referencing Professor John Gabrieli and Kathrin Karsay

This was only possible because I trusted myself, which is what I think resilience is. It's the ability to step outside of your comfort zone, to be okay with uncertainty, to avoid catastrophizing, and to not be in control. Having what feels like the entire world in the palm of our hand can easily trick us into feeling as though we should be in control of everything.

This can leave us feeling panicked when something happens that we weren't expecting. We automatically go into the 'fight, flight or freeze' mode, and our rational thinking switches off, leaving us in a state of fear that we work hard to avoid. However, it's often the avoidance of this that keeps us trapped in it, because we can't control everything in our life.

After I graduated from university, my brain simply shut down whenever I tried to apply for a job. I kept ending up on social media, scrolling through other people's lives, and spiralling into anxiety about my own. When I managed to get interviews, I had panic attacks and couldn't breathe. I stopped trusting myself and looked to other people to tell me what to do instead, as in 'N is for No'.

When I was 24, I decided I didn't want to live anymore. Ironically, reaching this point freed me to spend a week exactly how I wanted without worrying about the consequences, as I didn't think I'd be around to see them. I ate almond croissants for breakfast every day, ignored messages from people I didn't like, and chose to do only what I wanted to do each day. I realised that I'd accidentally started enjoying my life, instead of being scared of it.

During this period, I went to a mental health sharing circle set up by a charity called One Wave Is All It Takes. A man spoke about how he'd also felt suicidal, to the point that he'd left his partner in America and quit his job in search of trying to find a reason to live. A few weeks after leaving, he received a phone call telling him his girlfriend was murdered. Hearing this was the shock I needed to get me out of my pit of depression: **anybody could die at any time.** I realised my depression was making me feel as though my life was a never-ending prison sentence, but in reality, every second that I and the people I cared about were alive was a precious gift, as in 'T is for Time'. I stopped taking it all for granted and started living by the motto of 'I could be dead tomorrow'.

Living like this saw me stop overthinking every small decision and start living life on my terms. I moved to Byron Bay, started a blog which turned into *the Model Manifesto*, tried out jobs, spoke to people I didn't know who became lifelong friends, deleted my social media accounts as in 'Q is for Quitting', and chased every wild idea that came into my head. Two years later, I was on the cover of *the Times* and being interviewed on the *Lorraine* show about my best-selling book.

When I was writing it, I emailed world-famous people asking them if they wanted to be involved, and they said yes. I applied for jobs other people told me I had zero chance of getting, and was hired for them. I tried out things that seemed impossible, and they worked. I realised that the secret to success in life is resilience: the ability to withstand failure and rejection. For many of us, this will come with experience – when we experience pain so crushing we're not sure how we can survive, but somehow, we keep on going, and life gets better again.

Resilience is asking ourselves what the worst is that can happen, feeling the fear, and doing the things that scare us anyway. It's picking ourselves up and trying again. It's embracing the sad and difficult times as lessons – if nothing else, of what sadness means, so we can distinguish it from happiness. It's living our lives how we want to, instead of in fear.

Fear

As in 'C is for Content', we're more likely to see negative than positive news online, which shapes how we see the world. Although the world is objectively a much safer place today than it was 100 years ago, it's easy to believe that things have never been worse. For example, although the viral #metoo movement highlighted how commonplace sexual harassment and abuse of women and girls is, especially in the workplace, the fact that it's been shared so widely can make it feel as though it's happening right now.

Many of these stories happened a long time ago, but if we can read thousands of experiences in one hour, it's understandable to feel overwhelmed and hopeless about this issue. However, the fact that these stories are being shared is proof that things are changing, because many have clearly been silenced for many years. It's brilliant that the conversation is happening, but can still feel overwhelming to think of how far we still have to go when we try to engage with it online.

Social media can also stoke fear in us by comparisons with other people. I would often compare myself to other 'model activists' on Instagram, and convince myself my work was pointless because I didn't have as many followers as other people talking about these issues. It can set unrealistic bars of success for us to meet, as in 'P is for Perfectionism'.

The fears we have are often amplified on social media because this can make us believe that our opportunities are limited to our profiles. It allows us to obsess over our fears and stalk people more successful than us, and to reaffirm our beliefs that the world is a scary place. When we're stuck in a place of fear, we can't move forward: it's paralysing. The way to beat this, is to do it anyway. Once we fail at something, we realise it's not so bad after all – the world carries on spinning, and the pain fades, leaving a lesson behind for us to grow from next time.

Rejection

When I published *the Model Manifesto*, I made myself quite unwell by trying to control every aspect of it, as in 'P is for Perfectionism'. I was terrified of being wrong, which I assumed I most likely was, given that I was only a model and not an agency owner, accountant, psychiatrist, and so on! So I was very fortunate that many of these people spent their time in helping me with the book, which I hoped guarded me against negative feedback from all angles.

Obviously, it didn't. One of the people who kindly spent their time helping me and is thanked in the book even left a review online calling it 'victim tripe'. When I saw this, my heart dropped as I imagined all of the possible ways my life would now be ruined, imagining the headlines. However, the world simply doesn't care that much. Whether you're adored or hated by the public today, it'll probably be different tomorrow. You simply cannot please everybody, as in 'N is for No'.

You can be the ripest, juiciest peach in the world, and there will still be somebody out there who hates peaches. You can be as thin as I was at 18 (size 8), and still be called fat by a stranger on the street. You can be the most famous person in the world, and still be hated by people. There is simply no way to control what people think about you or what you do, so the best mode is to stay curious, don't take things too personally, and expect rejection.

My modelling career has prepared me very well for this, as I've been rejected more times than I can count, often straight to my face. I had no other choice but to cope with being insulted – what other options did I have? Argue back that I wasn't ugly? Insist I be booked for the job?

After one shoot I did, the client messaged my agency to say they weren't happy with me as a model, and refused to pay. I saw my pictures on their website the next day but they'd simply chopped the top of my face off! Another reshot a campaign I did on a different model after I'd done it, which I had to see every time I went into the tube station.

If I took every single comment personally, I probably wouldn't be able to get up in the mornings for fear of how offensive my appearance is.

If I dwelled on the amount of times I've been told to lose weight, I wouldn't be able to eat anything.

The secret to overcoming rejection is choosing what to believe. Whilst there's a difference between ignoring someone's boundaries and refusing to respect them, we can choose whether we want to take rejection on personally or not. For example, I reframed the negative reviews as a compliment and posted it on my own Instagram, as the fact that this person had bothered to go out of their way to leave such a mean review, must mean it's good enough to have hit a nerve!

As in 'K is for Kindness', people are not mean by nature. Despite this, social media opens us up to potential by an entire *world* of people we don't even know, and the key thing to remember is that although it might hurt, it doesn't really matter – it's not about us.

Failure

When we put ourselves in situations where we're afraid, such as taking a risk, or trying something again after failing, we tend to be vulnerable, as we're exposing ourselves to potential danger. Vulnerability can be related to the uncertainty, risk, and emotional exposure in being brave – researcher Brene Brown has an amazing Ted Talk on this.

For me, this is directly linked to how willing we are to release control over a situation. For example, after posting something on social media, I'd check it obsessively to monitor the immediate feedback, deleting and reposting if I didn't think this was good enough. This was keeping me trapped in the perfectionist model of fear, because I was still trying to control it.

In contrast, when I deleted my accounts, I released control over what people thought about me. I was scared of not being able to work anymore, but I needed to figure out how to live without this need of online validation for a while – and ironically worked more than ever!

Our society's emphasis, and especially the overload of self-help infographics on social media, can make us believe we 'should' be happy all the time – that this within our reach. However, it's ok to be upset, anxious, or disappointed. We should expect this, and embrace it, because it means we're human beings. We might be sad one day, and happy the next, and this all part of being alive.

Social media can trap us into not trying anything at all because we imagine everyone to care about what we do, but the most important realisation I've had is that nobody really cares. If I try something and fail, most people won't notice. Worst case scenario, someone might rub it in my face. Once they've done that, they go on living their life. If I try something and succeed, most people won't really care. Some might be impressed for a day or like my online post about it, but then they go on living their life. The only way we learn is by trying, and experiencing all the complex emotions that come along with this.

If you can imagine something, you can do it. Those wild ideas you're afraid of trying are what will make you happy, because you'll know you tried. You won't get to the end of your life with a secret diary filled with brilliant ideas, but you'll have a squiggly, vibrant line of dots that all add up to make your colourful life. Please don't give that up to look in a screen – there's much more to life than social media.

Don't be afraid of failure or negative feelings – embrace them. These are what will direct you on a happier path. It's impossible to summarise the complexities of emotions, vulnerabilities and fears into a social media post, so focus on feeling these things in real life, instead of distracting yourself online.

Tips

- Make a 'resilience list' of the tough times you've had, and things you've done that you didn't think you'd be able to do.

- What would you do if you had 5 years left to live? How about 1 week? What's holding you back from doing the things you want to do right now?
- What would you do if you know you couldn't fail? Try to identify one small step you could take to actually *do* this thing right now.
- Remember that no one really cares about what you do or don't do. Anyone that can be bothered to make any kind of negative comment clearly has their own problems, as in 'K is for Kindness' – don't take them on yourself!
- Try out one small action outside of your comfort zone, such as trying out a new sport, or going to a networking event by yourself.
- If you feel scared by this, can you question the thoughts behind it? What are you believing about the situation, and what proof do you have for this? What proof do you have for other, perfectly reasonable explanations?
- If you're feeling worried, ask yourself what the worst case scenario is in any situation. Imagine a ditch, with this scenario at the bottom. Now imagine a ladder out of the ditch, with each step of what you'd do next. This is life: even if we ended up being 'cancelled' online, our real life would go on. We always have options, even if fear clouds our vision sometimes.
- Try to ground yourself, as in 'U is for Unreal', and identify how a situation will feel in 1 month, 6 months, and 1 year.

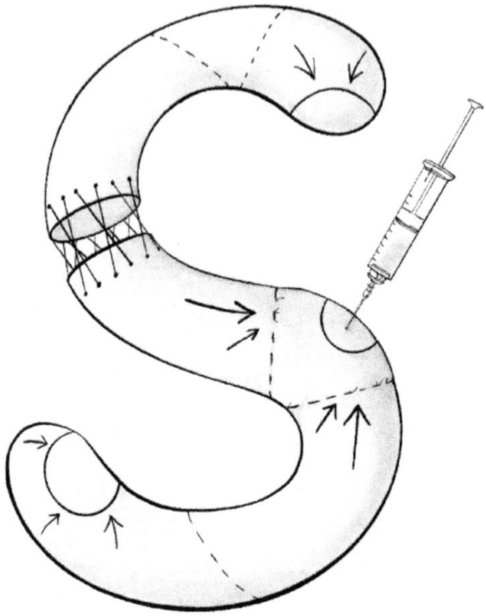

is for Surgery

S is for Surgery

Did you know?

- Researchers have identified a 'slim-thick' body ideal inspired by Kim Kardashian's hourglass figure to be more harmful for women's body image than Kate Moss' ultra-thin frame.[35]

When our grandparents were growing up, they'd see as many 'beautiful' women in one year as we see in one day. They might have seen a movie star on a poster, but they wouldn't have been bombarded with an endless stream of photos of them from the second they woke up to when they went to sleep. Our grandparents didn't have filters showing them how they could look with a different nose or jaw. There was no pressure to post photographs of themselves on the internet – it didn't even exist!

Many years ago, a model I worked with regularly at a top e-commerce brand was crying hysterically because she'd been dropped. The reason wasn't because she'd put on weight (this same brand made me 'tone up' for 3 months), but because she'd had lip filler. They said they could not hire models who'd had cosmetic surgery – the practice of having their appearance physically changed by medical procedures.

This seemed unfair given that the company often flew in new models from Brazil who'd talk about the procedures they'd had to achieve the precise dimensions of their bodies! It was also ironic given that

---

[35] Jonathan Chadwick, 'Kim Kardashian's hourglass figure is more harmful for women's body image than Kate Moss' thin frame, study claims', *Mail Online*, 25 January 2022. Accessed 20 February 2022. www.dailymail.co.uk/sciencetech/article-10440489/Kim-Kardashians-hourglass-figure-harmful-body-image-study-says.html

their maternity models weren't pregnant, but were strapping on a fake baby bump, with no disclosure of this to the customer.

Today, this brand, along with many other 'fast-fashion' retailers are filled with pictures of models who have had cosmetic surgery. Bluntly, having surgery wasn't in fashion back then – but it is now. A decade ago, it would have been a shameful secret, but today it's become as normalised as getting a manicure, presented as a 'self-care routine'.

Fixing ourselves

I was 21 when someone first suggested I get Botox because of my 'forehead wrinkles'. I'd already convinced myself I was too old to be a model at that age, and this made me feel even more insecure. However, I knew that once I'd started, I wouldn't be able to stop, and objectively speaking it seemed ridiculous to have Botox at age 21! After spending lots of money I didn't have on skincare products instead, a facialist told me they weren't wrinkles - I just needed to drink water.

In comparison, a woman told me how she was offered a free consultation whilst waiting for a friend having a cosmetic procedure done in a clinic. As in 'B is for Beauty', she had her photograph taken, before being shown her face blown-up on a giant screen in front of her. The clinicians had drawn big red circles around parts of her face she'd never thought about before, such as her jawline, and showed her how they could 'fix' these. Then they showed her what she 'could' look like instead.

Needless to say, she left the clinic much poorer and unhappier that she had been whilst innocently walking in to wait for her friend. The woman had never had any insecurities about her face before, but left with a whole new list of reasons to hate herself and spend more money, paying for procedures she'd never even heard of before that day. A similar thing can happen to models -I know one who had a client had make her squeeze into a size 0 dress and circle the areas she needed to 'tone up' in red, sending this to her agency. People are not objects, and it's impossible to mould ourselves in this way, not that we need to in the first place!

However, having the suggestion made to us that we could be a better version of ourselves makes us believe there is something that needs fixing. Every time I look at the photos on my phone, it makes suggestions to me of how it can 'fix' the photos. Everything from social media apps to video conferencing software has built in 'beauty enhancer' tools that make me look like a completely different person. These tools do not make us look any more beautiful – they just make us look less human.

You are not broken, and there is nothing to fix. You are simply a human being, with a face that moves, a body that contains organs, a bunch of cells and magic blended together. When we start believing we need to fix ourselves somehow, we can't stop, because there was never anything wrong in the first place – but this doesn't stop us from trying.

Cosmetic Surgery

Every day, I learn about new procedures people are having done to their body. Last week I met a woman who'd had a procedure to chemically curl her eyelashes, which brought back painful memories of seeing models have half their eyelashes chopped off by make up artists during shows! This woman still had her eyelashes, but one side had become uncurled, meaning she looked rather unusual.

Another showed me how she'd had a procedure to layer her teeth with the material used in fillings, almost like having fake nails stuck on. A teenager I spoke to recently told me how she wanted to have Botox as soon as possible as a 'preventative measure'. Another showed me the world of 'Brazilian Butt Lifts', where fat is moved from one part of the body to another. A friend explained how she was saving up thousands of pounds to have her 'eye-bags' eradicated with surgery, but she'd never tell anyone about it.

As a model, I've been sent castings that deliberately seek out people with no surgery to sell a procedure. Legally, they have to do 'something', so the casting said the job would only involve a glossing treatment instead of doing any actual injections, but it would've advertised a total transformation as a result of a surgical procedure I wouldn't have had. There's no way of telling what's real or not, unless you're actually on the job. Nowadays, when I model for large companies, I have to sign declarations confirming the product was actually used on the day.

This is the point we've come to in advertising – but not on social media. Social media is ultimately a business platform, where we are being marketed to, but there is absolutely zero regulation of how trustworthy these products are, as in 'M is for Money'. Just look at how many 'influencers' are promoting detox teas and juices, or magical 'remedies' that give them the look they've completely invented using digital tools like filters and photoshop.

The impact of this is standards being set that simply do not exist. Just like an adult woman trying to look like the 13-year-old version of me in *Vogue*, this is impossible unless she can reverse puberty – or surgically mould her body. She will never look like the girl in the magazines, because she is an adult woman, and even that girl doesn't exist. I didn't look like me in *Vogue*, I looked like a gawky teenager who was bullied for being ugly!

Social media not only presents these images to us but pressurises us to step into them ourselves. It gives us filters like 'Perfect Face!' which will give us an entirely new nose, free of charge. It takes away the pores in our skin and gives us bright white teeth and eyes, which is simply not real. However, if this is all we see, it's easy to believe that it should be achievable by any means necessary.

It can also seem like we *should* look like these fake versions of ourselves online, because that's what we see around us. For example, the number of labiaplasty operations have risen up to 45% year on year, as the 'world's fastest-growing cosmetic procedure'.[36] As in 'X is for X-rated', if pornography only shows Barbie-like genital areas on women, and social media shows micro-thong-string-bikinis that seem to confirm the same, it's natural to think that a vagina area 'should' basically be as invisible as possible. In reality, there all different kinds of shapes, sizes, colours, and asymmetries – and believe it or not, hair does grow naturally down there for everyone!

Having cosmetic surgery can impact the sensations we can feel in these areas, and some practitioners have compared labiaplasty (cosmetic surgery to reduce the labia in size – skin either side of the vaginal opening) to female genital mutilation. Needless to say, whichever surgery you have, it will HURT! It also tends to be extremely expensive, with some procedures costing thousands of pounds.

Even if we have surgery to change how we look, the initial effect will not last. This is the point – to keep you going back for more. Surgery might be able to freeze your forehead temporarily, but eventually reality will kick back in, and your face will move when you talk again. You are a human being, not a digital avatar. The procedure you want isn't not even going to do what it's intended to do, because you will need to go back for more and more, just like a drug. It will become normal, and you'll be onto the next thing.

The surgery treadmill

As in 'Z is for Zen', Body Dysmorphia Disorder is a mental health condition involving an obsessive preoccupation with what we believe are 'flaws' about our appearances. Most models I know have this, due to a career involving comparing ourselves of people that look very similar to us, but just a tiny bit more 'beautiful' in some way.

---

[36] Katie Forster, 'Labiaplasty: vaginal surgery 'world's fastest-growing cosmetic procedure', says plastic surgeons', *the Independent*, 12 July 2017. Accessed 20 February 2022.

When I finally lost the weight that my agency wanted me to lose, as in 'D is for Disordered Eating', they told me to lose some more. They also booked me a £400 hair appointment where my hair was dyed brown, without me knowing. A woman was appointed to take me clothes shopping, to pick out what I should wear – at a cost of over £300 to me. I was even instructed on how to greet the agents themselves with an 'air-kiss'. When I didn't do this, I was told off.

This is because once you start trying to 'fix' yourself (or someone else, as in my case), it becomes very difficult to stop. I don't know at what point this agency would have accepted me for who I was, because fortunately I realised it was never going to end and plucked up the courage to leave by myself. As in 'P is for Perfectionism', there is simply no definable 'end goal' – you will never know when you're done.

Surgery gives us an illusion of control over our physical bodies, but this doesn't stop the mind running the show. When we're unhappy with how we look, we can tinker with our outsides all we want, but we won't be happy until we sort the insides out. If our brain is fixated on a 'problem' such as a specific feature of ours, changing that feature won't necessarily make the problem go away – we will just find something new to obsess over. This is how surgery can easily become addictive.

Whilst it would have been great to have waved a magic wand over myself as an 18 year old to look how this agency wanted me to look, I still would have felt as ugly as ever. I'd never felt more self-conscious as when I was trying to be this Barbie doll version of myself that they wanted me to be. When we figure out how to feel good for ourselves, this radiates outwards.

Trends & Black Markets

A few years ago, I had my teeth whitened via an app that gave models free things in return for social media posts. Even though this didn't last very long at all (and hurt a LOT!), when I posted about it online, I had a lot of interest from my followers. This is because I normalised doing a procedure to myself that other people could do, just the popular 'what I eat in a day' videos. I was showing that despite being a model in magazines, I was on the same treadmill as everybody else, seemingly paying money and undergoing procedures in trying to make myself more attractive.

In comparison, Kim Kardashian has never publicly confirmed having cosmetic surgery, and even outright denied it. She's instead put the significant differences in her current appearance to how it was 10 years ago, down to make up or lighting, whilst selling her own range of 'shapewear' lingerie. If she'd confirmed having surgery, this would undermine her entire business built on convincing people they could possibly look like her, if they bought enough of her products, as in 'M is for Money'.

The Kardashians' success in being famous for being famous has had a ripple effect through the rest of our society. Impossible body proportions that are simply unachievable for most people are now held up as the ideal. Unlike the terrible 'size 0' trend, we're aware this isn't theoretically achievable through severe dieting, as in 'E is for Eating', because it involves moulding parts of our bodies to be bigger and smaller, which is just impossible to do naturally, no matter how hard we try.

This leaves us very vulnerable to cosmetic surgery adverts promising a 'quick fix' of achieving a Kardashian-style body. A recent investigation highlighted how practitioners with no medical qualifications were targeting women and girls on social media in trying to persuade them to have unlicensed cosmetic surgical procedures, finding that many people who had had these 'black market' treatments ended up permanently scarred or disfigured.[37]

---

[37] Charlotte Wace and Paul Morgan-Bentley, ''Black market' Botox scars women for life', *the Sunday Times*, 2 February 2022. Accessed 20 February 2022. www.thetimes.co.uk/article/black-market-botox-scars-women-for-life-khr5g2bnk

This is an entirely unregulated practice of deliberately targeting vulnerable people on social media to prey on their insecurities in extremely dangerous ways.

You are beautiful as you are, and ultimately, we are all bags of jelly wandering around this earth. We're all different, and that's what makes us all uniquely ourselves, because we've been given these miraculous bodies that do everything they can to keep us alive, which is easy to take for granted. Try a process of radical gratitude instead of judging yourself – there's so much more to life than the proportions of your body.

Tips

- Are there any parts of your body you'd like to change? If so, can you ask yourself why? Where has this thought come from?

- Can you compare this body part to another part of your body, such as your elbows or ankles? Ultimately, it's all part of the same package, but we – or society - attaches different meaning to different parts. Imagine if an alien came down and saw us all obsessing over the dimensions of our hips, or how much we weigh on the planet!

- Try to identify what beliefs underpin your negative feelings about your body, and work through them with a therapist. You could also question them, and get very specific: what practical impact would changing something have?

- If you notice a negative thought about your appearance, try to ask yourself whether it's a useful thought to have. You don't have to look at yourself, other people do!

- Identify how you want to feel about your body, and focus on the parts you're grateful for. What would your life be like if they disappeared overnight?

- Imagine a child or a friend saying the negative thoughts you have about yourself, about themselves. How would you feel?
- Try to replace negative thoughts with gratitude, remembering happy experiences you've had in your body, such as going on a fun holiday.
- Avoid looking at content that presents unrealistic beauty standards, if you can, such as unfollowing people who use filters – and try not to use these yourself!
- Try to do activities that help you to appreciate your body. This could include finding a sport you enjoy, or simply taking a few minutes each day to feel the different parts of your body.
- Try a life drawing class – it's very helpful to see real human bodies, and acknowledge how beautiful they are! Body Love Sketch Club have some incredible classes.
- If you want to have surgery, take your time to think about this. I am neither for or against surgery, but it's important to know why you're doing it, what you're doing it for, and to be realistic about the outcomes.

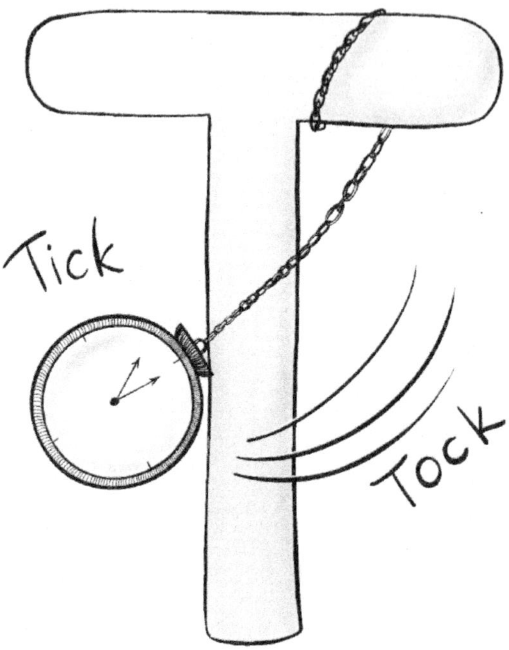

is for Time

T is for Time

Did you know?

- It takes over 23 minutes to regain your focus when you're interrupted by distractions whilst trying to focus on something else, such as checking your social media feeds.[38]

Do you feel like you're in control of your own time? Technology can give us the illusion of this, by allowing us to fast-forward videos or voice notes, or skip to the end of books, but ultimately, it takes our time away.

Today, we're all accessible 24 hours a day. So much information is being pelted at us that our brains are struggling to keep up by going faster and faster, until we crash and burn out. When we're getting hundreds of emails every day, how do we find the time to read them all? How can we keep up with voice notes and podcasts and music? How do we keep up with all our friends' lives, and our own? If you're feeling like there's simply not enough time in the day, you're not alone.

Having ADHD is strongly linked with problems related to time management, because our brains seem to know only two senses of time: 'now', and 'not now'. We struggle with making decisions about the future, remembering the past, managing our emotions, and thinking through possible options. In summary, we can struggle with 'delayed gratification': giving up something in the present to work towards something we know will be good for us in the future.

---

[38] Brian Solis, 'Our digital malaise: distraction is costing us more than we think' | LSE Business Review, 19 April 2019. Accessed 17 March 2022. Referencing Gloria Mark, University of California.

For example, we'd rather eat croissants for breakfast today than porridge, because we struggle to think about our 'future selves'. If we're in an intensely focused state, it can be difficult to disengage from this, because we're not sure when it'll come again! We might say 'yes' automatically, having to cancel later, as in 'N is for No'. This can result in serious challenges including literally managing our lives, relationships, work, emotions, self-esteem, and impulsivity.

Unfortunately, this is how social media and screens are training us all to be. We're in the world of instant hits of gratification, of pleasure today rather than tomorrow, of being used to being able to see whatever we want, when we want. We're used to having the world of knowledge at our fingertips, and knowing the answers to questions within seconds, as in 'R is for Resilience'. We're being conditioned to see seemingly unlimited choices of how to spend our time every time we look at our phones and can't properly decide what to do with it.

We're being tricked into thinking we should be able to do everything, which leaves us doing nothing, feeling overwhelmed and guilty. If our phones are giving us the equivalent of junk food stimulation throughout the day, it can be very difficult to think about the future and work towards long-term goals. What we want out of life is replaced by what we're presented on social media as 'aesthetic', as in 'O is for Objectification'.

To overcome the challenge of trying to have it all, we try to do everything. For example, we take photos of experiences we want to enjoy such as concerts or holidays to 'enjoy it later', or 'remember it'. By experiencing something through a phone, we're unable to enjoy it, and becoming hooked on the junk food version of delayed gratification by trying to drag out experiences, feeling the main 'enjoyment' from when we post about it on social media. As a result, we end up replacing any positive feelings from an experience with the highs of social media, as in 'V is for Validation'.

Distractions & procrastination

The way I managed to learn entire years' worth of subjects for my exams in months was by having the passwords to my social media accounts, as in 'Q is for Quitting'. Whenever we go on our phones with a certain intention, such as to open a message, we are distracted in a clever, subconscious way by programming. More red notification bubbles tempt us into opening them, other apps taunt us with the need to check them 'just in case' we're missing out on something, and the shiny colours and over-stimulation of many different options diverts us from our original intention, as in 'A is for Algorithms'. Just like we might forget what we're talking about mid-way through a conversation, our phones can easily distract us from what we were planning to do.

Take it from someone with ADHD – it's impossible to do anything properly if we're trying to do everything! My brain can often feel like it has 150 tabs open at the same time, which makes it very difficult to try and concentrate on anything. When we lose the ability to focus, we lose the ability to experience life properly.

The ultimate impact of this is on you and your time. When we get distracted and fall into a scrolling vortex, that can last for hours, we are effectively having our time *stolen*. It might not feel like that, because we may enjoy the cute animal videos, but if you were actually trying to complete a project, for example, which has now become much harder, this is stopping you from doing what you wanted to do.

Commitment

The time as I write this is 6:26am. I have already spent over 20 minutes of my morning reading about celebrities and negative news, which has been time I wanted to spend writing this book. This is despite having zero social media apps on my phone, most news websites blocked, no Instagram, Facebook or TikTok, no internet connection on my laptop, and no notifications!

To complete something that we truly want to get done, we must fight for it. We have to choose to spend our limited time in certain ways, accepting that we simply can't do everything at once. We need to dedicate time, break down individual tasks, set deadlines, and hold ourselves accountable. We have to admit defeat to distractions and simply remove them in order to avoid procrastination. For me, this has involved waking up at 6am every day to try and finish this book – not because I even have a book deal or external deadline, but because I feel that it's important. If my experiences can help someone else, they're worth sharing.

Committing to something means prioritizing it over other things, which can feel very difficult to do in a world of unlimited potential opportunities – but I recommend starting with one goal. Start with completing one thing that means something to you, and watch your self-esteem build. Just make sure you know when you're finished!

Faster doesn't mean better

When I studied law, every week I was assigned to read judgments of cases and textbook material that were hundreds of pages long, which I never did. I just went on Wikipedia and memorised the summary. Driven by fear of having learned nothing throughout the year, I'd hyper-focus on these summaries before my exams and cram them into my brain, graduating with very good marks.

Although I got the degree, I felt I had learned nothing of great significance, and I had graduated with no idea of how to cope in the 'real world'. I was crippled by imposter syndrome and thought I was too stupid to ever get a job, believing I'd somehow cheated in my degree by simply being unable to learn like everybody else. It was only when I was diagnosed with ADHD years later that I managed to have compassion for myself and appreciate how to use these strengths in ways that are more meaningful to me!

However, the point of this is that doing things quickly, even if they seem to be done 'well', can remove the meaning behind it. What's the point of getting A's in exams if you haven't learned anything? We can send 100 messages a day, but do we really know what we're saying in these messages? Audiobooks allow us to listen all day, but are we really taking anything in?

Communication

When the way we process information is sped up, so is our communication. As in 'F is for Friendship', we can talk to seemingly lots of people, but feel more alone than ever. Compare sending a post card to sending a voice note - although sending a post card might have less information in it, it's meaningful because someone has taken the time to think of us whilst they were on holiday. They've taken time out of their break to buy us a card and stamp, hand write us a note, and to post this to our address from a different country. It might arrive weeks after they return, but this is what makes it so lovely.

There's nothing quite like receiving a handwritten letter in the post – I'd strongly recommend sending thank you letters if you want to leave a good impression on someone, such as after an interview!

In comparison, we might be able to easily send lots of voice notes lasting several minutes long or ping off lots of emails, but we might not say very much. It's easy to mindlessly speak into our phones, feeling as though we're giving updates on our lives, but much more difficult to listen to a person narrating their lives to us. I had friends where we'd voice note each other constantly, but never actually spoke on the phone, or saw each other in real life. When we send a voice note, we're also sending an implication that the person take time out of their day to listen to us and reply to everything we've said, which might be quite a lot!

This can lead to us speeding up voice notes to listen to them, or not being able to properly respond to everything someone says, because we simply can't remember it. Our email inbox might have 1000 unread messages, but we might feel like nobody really wants to talk to us. When we ping off responses to keep up the dopamine hits of ticking people off like items on a 'to do' list, it leaves us feeling empty, because we're losing connection.

Memory

If it feels like your memory is getting worse, that may be because it's being outsourced to technology. When we're using Facebook to keep track of birthdays, Instagram to keep track of our best moments, or our online calendars to remember our schedules, we're delegating the parts of our brains that need to remember this to social media. Just like our leg muscles would need retraining if we lay in bed for a month, if we stop using our memory, it becomes weaker.

If we overload our days with so much information, especially when this mainly happens through a screen, it becomes much harder to remember it all. Our past experiences and memories make up who we are today, both the good and the bad. For us to be able to truly know ourselves, or develop as people, we need to be able to remember our past and our values. If all we have to remember our past is a glossy highlights reel, we're at risk of forgetting the important lessons that more difficult times have taught us, and falsely believing the present reality is worse than the past.

When our brains are moving so quickly, we must consciously train ourselves in patience. This ultimately requires us to trust ourselves in being able to manage our time and energy appropriately so that we don't burn out, implementing strategies to do so that are not rooted in technology. The problem with using technology to manage our time, tell us what to do, or be our memory, is that it is biased – it wants us to keep spending our time on it. Whilst technology can help remind us of certain things, it shouldn't replace our memories all together – or our time.

The luxury of time

After I graduated from university and felt lost about what to 'do' with my life, I became very depressed, leading to feeling suicidal. Fortunately, I realised that my mind was tricking me into believing I had endless years to fill, which is a luxury, because time isn't guaranteed to any of us.

We could all literally drop dead at any second, and so could the people we love. We're all dying, because death is the only guarantee in life – and that's what makes it worth living. The fact that we've got limited time makes it special and frees us to do what we want, because we might not be here tomorrow.

Our modern world can both make us feel as though we don't have enough time to do all the things we want to do, and too much. Social media can trick us into taking it for granted, believing that we can enjoy things 'later' by posting about them online, whilst also preventing us from being able to properly think about our long-term future. Distractions can knock us off track from working towards what we want in life, sucking up our time in meaningless activities that can often leave us feeling worse off.

Your engagement is valuable, not just to the companies that are paying for it, but ultimately to you, because this is essentially how you're spending your time here on this earth. Who is profiting from how you're spending your time?

Time is an incredibly valuable gift to all of us. You have inherent worth just by being alive – think of all the chance encounters that have had to happen for you to actually exist! If you are struggling, remind yourself that you are here for a reason. You matter. Your time matters. It belongs to you – not your phone. It is your greatest luxury in life to choose how to spend it – don't let this be stolen from you without even realising until it's too late. If you're feeling overwhelmed with how to best use your time, just take a breath and remember how fortunate you are to be alive.

Tips

- The average person has a life expectancy of approximately 4000 weeks. How are you spending yours?

- If you can, track your time for a day. Set yourself hourly reminders throughout the day and record what you do throughout, noting down when you start a new task, or get distracted.

- If you were to die at 100 years old, what would you want your epitaph to read? What impact do you want to leave on the world? This doesn't have to be writing books or leaving a shrine of perfect selfies, but how do you want to make people feel? What do you want to experience in your life – not for social media, but to truly experience?

- Write down all the experiences you want to have, and pick one thing at a time. Imagine these things are fish in a river, and you can only cook one at a time (metaphorically!) – you can always come back to the other ones, but if you try to do them all at once, they'll all die. What fish do you want to pick first? Can you make a commitment to doing this with the limited time you have? If you're not sure, can you identify what you care about in life, and simply commit to living by your 'values' each day?

- Can you assess the 'opportunity cost' of your time, and identify what you are choosing to 'miss out' on? For example, by writing this book I'm missing out on being able to watch television and see people I care about, but this is a temporary choice that I'm consciously aware of.

- How can you think of your time more in terms of happiness than productivity? What do you care about in life?

- Try to take breaks to recharge every day, and to plan out what you do and don't want to spend your time doing.

- Keep a journal and write about your days. This validates your own experiences and imprints who you are into your memory, because you're spending time on yourself, with no objectification or expectations on what you might write – you're simply living your life for you, which is the greatest luxury of all.

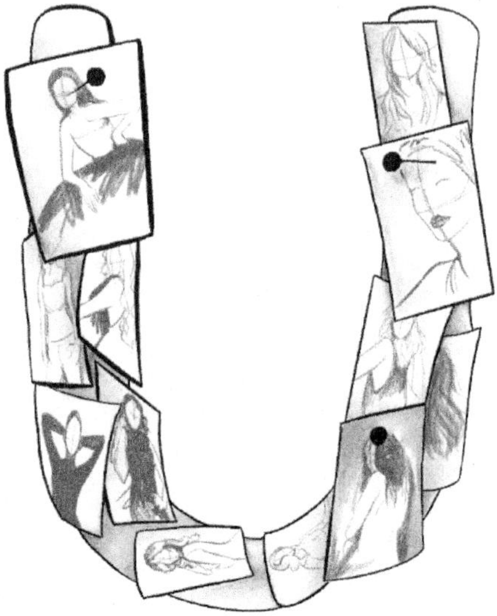

is for Unreal

U is for Unreal

Did you know?

- The number of 'deepfake' videos, a type of media created with artificial intelligence that can make it look as though a person is in a video, have doubled every six months since observations started in December 2019.[39] As of September 2019, 96% of deepfake videos online were pornographic. [40]

The problem with the online world is that it is not real, so it's always going to leave us unsatisfied. We'll never be truly happy with a half-life lived throughout a world that doesn't really exist, because we're not algorithms – we're human beings. We have senses to experience the world around us with, emotions that make us feel alive, and bodies that develop over time. We grow older, and eventually die, but this is part of what makes being a human so amazing – we're not here forever, so we might as well enjoy what we've got.

When we live through a screen, these aspects of being human can be ignored, numbed, dulled, or distorted. It's easy to convince ourselves we've got the entire world at our fingertips, so why bother experiencing it at all? When our minds are so overstimulated with technology, our real life can seem dull in comparison – but it's not. The unrealistic standards we see online can become what we set ourselves to meet in reality, but this is simply not possible, because they don't exist.

---

[39] Vilius Petkauskas, 'Report: number of deepfakes double every six months' | CyberNews, 3 May 2021. Accessed 17 March 2022.
[40] Rob Toews, 'Deepfakes Are Going To Wreak Havoc On Society. We Are Not Prepared.' (forbes.com). Accessed 17 March 2022.

Appearance

As seen throughout this book, social media is distorting our standards of beauty to be something that doesn't even exist at all. The ultimate 'aspiration' would be something that tricks our mind into thinking we should be able to achieve it, regardless of it being impossible. When we can see our bodies morphed within seconds by filters, or are bombarded with images of people that have had cosmetic surgery, we can easily set these as our new standards to meet in reality.

Although these are objectively not achievable, social media tricks us into believing they are, with videos such as 'what I eat in a day'. As in 'C is for Content', there is zero regulation or oversight of this content, and we can simply be being lied to and manipulated. When we hate our bodies simply for existing as they are, this can leave us feeling out of control and desperate to 'fix' ourselves in some way. However, we will just never, ever look like our virtual avatar selves in real life, because these have been edited in ways that are impossible to achieve or sustain in reality.

I know how drastically a make-up artist can change my face on a photoshoot, but I also know how many years they've had to train for and sit through hours of being made up. This reminds me not to compare myself to this 'fixed' version of me, because I know how difficult it is to achieve in reality. I know that even with this professional expertise, I might still look 'bad' on camera if the lighting, styling or posing isn't right. I often see the 100 bad pictures a photographer has to take before they find 1 that is acceptable. However, most people do not have this experience – they simply see the final product, and assume I look like that all of the time, which I very rarely do!

Just as we don't compare ourselves to literal objects such as chairs, we shouldn't compare ourselves to concepts that don't even exist, especially when these are designed to manipulate us into feeling bad about ourselves.

Success

Social media gives us a highlights reel which can feel like a form of control, by focusing on our successes and achievements. We don't tend to post the average day-to-day things in our lives, such as the projects we're working on at school or work, which can give the illusion of everybody having fun, exciting and successful lives all the time.

This is even more obvious when we compare the 'metrics' of these posts, as in 'J is for Jealousy'. It's easy to ignore any successes that aren't visually pleasing or worthy of being posted online for some reason, and only focus on 'pretty' ones, such as going on a luxury holiday. This can also lead us to believe that we can only be happy if we're 'successful', moulding the way we see our own lives to seek out opportunities to post things online.

When we live online, everything meshes into one experience. From playing a videogame where you're driving a high-speed car, to reading celebrity gossip, or watching explicit content, as in 'X is for X-rated', it all blends into the same numb feeling. After the initial high of trying something out for the first time, it will simply become normal, with no variety between experiences except those that bring out the most extreme reactions in us. We're fortunate to have a range of senses to experience the world with, including taste, touch, smell, sound and sight – why limit yourself to one dimension?

It's important to remember that most of what we see online is fake – from the number of followers, likes, and comments a person has, to the wonderfully happy relationship they seem to be in. When we brand ourselves, as in 'O is for Objectification', we can easily lose touch with reality, which always comes with a complex range of emotions and situations. Literally no one is happy 100% of the time, because we are human. As in 'P is for Perfectionism', life isn't always good, and everybody experiences failures and rejections, but they just don't always post about it.

Relationships

Social media can it seem as though everybody is popular and well-liked except us. It can trick us into constantly checking up on our connections with other people, as we're given access to the inner worlds of many people that we know in real life. Ironically, it can also make us feel as though we have almost too many connections at the same time.

Virtual friends are not our real friends. I knew people who had hundreds of thousands of Instagram followers, with odd lives of being world-famous on their phones, but essentially 'normal' in reality. If we're constantly being pelted with messages and notifications, this can lead us to feel as though we're always indebted to other people who we don't even know.

As in 'L is for Love', it's very easy to build an entire online persona and relationship that is completely different to how things are in reality. As much as we might want to be different people, creating an online persona isn't the way to do this – reality will always catch up with us in the end, because that's the world we live in – not the virtual one.

The relationships we see online are often nowhere near as good as they look, especially if they seem to revolve largely around social media. People who genuinely care about each other don't need to prove it to the entire world. Ironically, this is more likely to be a sign of insecurity!

Knowledge

The virtual world is making our brains go faster and faster, pelting us with endless information and updates. Have you ever just switched between lots of different apps, not actually going on them, but just seeing if there's anything new? Compare this to reading a book! It might seem counter-intuitive to learn how to do maths instead of using a calculator, for example, but that's the point: to be able to *learn*. When we stop using our brains to solve problems, they become weaker, and we give up our autonomy to companies profiting from us to tell us the answer.

Googling something isn't the same as using a calculator, because Google is a profit-making technology corporation, not a black-and-white object. The more information we're hit with, the more difficult it becomes to prioritise between it, which means we're more likely to go for the first available answer – even if this has been paid to rank first in the search engine. It can be hard to care when we're on the hunt for answers as quickly as possible, in comparison to the days of having to search for answers in a library!

This overload of information isn't knowledge – it's overwhelming. We're unable to process or prioritize it and may find it difficult to understand what is 'real' or not. When we stop being able to understand information and think clearly, life can seem pretty meaningless – why bother putting the work in for anything if we're so used to having immediate gratification? The more we live in this illusion of knowledge, the more we feel like imposters, trapped by the luxuries we think we have.

Choices

Living like this disconnects you from reality, and from yourself. It becomes very hard to figure out who *you* are, or what you want, because it's so easy to ask Google. When we're only able to concentrate for a few seconds before being distracted by something else, we can't think about the long term, because our sense of time is distorted. I recently had my hair done on a modelling job for 10 *hours*, all for a 30 second TikTok video to be filmed! How are we supposed to have future goals if we're living for content that's already old news as soon as it's posted?

Living in this world can also make us more impulsive, chasing whatever idea we've had that day after being influenced by our screens. From booking holidays to buying products, trying out new recipes to dangerous pranks, it becomes harder to make a distinction between these types of decisions. As a result, we're being driven to always want more, where settling on one choice in a world of limitless choices feels impossible.

Social media stops us from feeling our own emotions, a tempting and constantly accessible way of numbing ourselves from reality by scrolling. It's only when we come offline, back into our messy, imperfect realities, that we feel bad – and so log back on to search for ways to make us feel better. It makes us intolerable to pain, boredom, or real life – the cause is not the solution.

The only thing that will truly help us to overcome these feelings, is the conscious choosing of reality. It's choosing to experience our lives as they are, to be bored, to reconnect with ourselves. The virtual, unreal world might be fun to hop into every so often, but it shouldn't overtake our real one. Our brains are very resilient and can adapt back to reality if we consciously take the steps to make this happen.

There's nothing more rewarding in life than living it, along with the messy, complicated experiences that make us human. Just like we can't know what happiness is without sadness, our lives are not supposed to be airbrushed to perfection highlights reels where everything feels exactly the same. We all have the power to decide follow what interests us, what we want to do, and who we want to be – don't let this be taken away from you.

<u>**Tips**</u>

- How does the thought of spending a day off your phone make you feel? Can you give it a go?
- Spot the moments that you automatically reach for your phone. Is it when you're bored, or alone?
- Test your willpower muscles, such as by not picking up your phone when you get a notification, or only checking your emails once a day. Every time you consciously decide to do

something else rather than automatically go on your phone, you are training your brain in self-control.

- The next time you receive a message, simply notice what happens to your body, feeling the experience of anticipation. Notice how you feel (usually anti-climactic!), and what you automatically want do afterwards, and try doing something different.
- Get an alarm clock and setting a later time in the morning for when you will first check your phone – not the most instagrammable #morningroutine, but a million times better in reality!
- Try out this simple exercise a few times a day: notice 5 things that you can see, 4 things you can hear, 3 things you can feel, 2 things you can smell, and 1 thing you can taste. If you notice that your brain feels over-stimulated or isn't sure what to do next at any point, just do this exercise.
- If you feel uncomfortable at any point, or any of the anxious emotions that you've maybe been trying to avoid, simply allow them to be there. This will help you to process them properly, instead of stuffing them into a mental cupboard, where they'll inevitably explode. Try to make a list of the things you're grateful for in that moment, and feel the feelings eventually pass.
- Try to consciously be bored, which is vital for our creativity and resilience. For example, walk down the street in silence, instead of playing music, or give yourself periods of time where you do nothing but look out of a window. It feels completely opposite to what we've been conditioned to think of as 'productive', but you are strengthening your brain.
- Make your screens as boring as possible, such as by setting a black and white screen, and turning off the notifications

completely. By removing the 'junk food' dopamine highs, we're strengthening our ability to feel them in reality – like skipping fast food to properly enjoy a healthy, nutritious meal.

- Identify a 'grounding activity' to do, which is completely separate to the virtual world and makes you feel happy, such as cooking or painting.

- Try to choose something else to do instead of going on your phone as a replacement activity, such as journaling first thing in the morning or before you go to sleep.

- Spend time with people in real life, with no technology present.

- Try to notice 3 things per day that you feel grateful for, especially when you're feeling tempted to go on your phone. Try to consciously experience whatever you're doing in any second, feeling what it's like to have that experience, and think of how lucky you are to be able to do it.

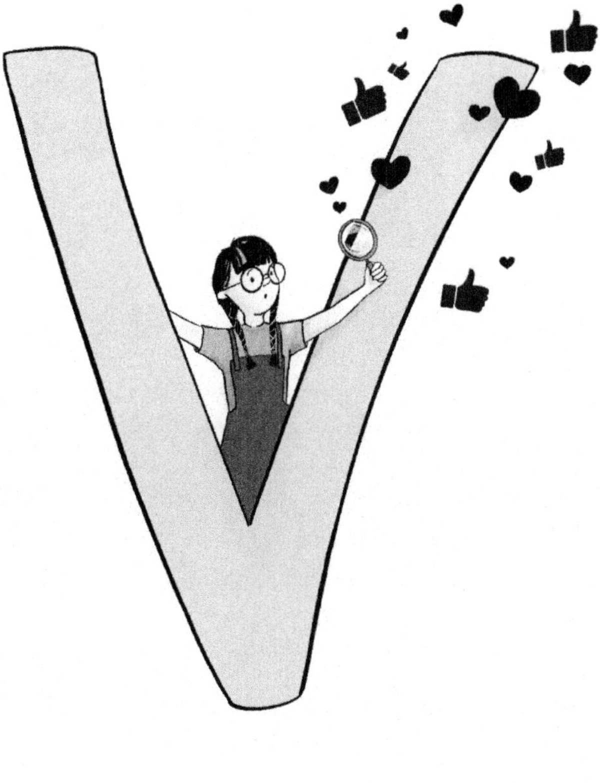

is for Validation

V is for Validation

Did you know?

- Simply not getting enough validation on social media has been proven to increase depression and anxiety, especially for adolescents. Not getting enough 'likes' causes them to reduce their feelings of self-worth. [41]

For me, the most addictive part of social media is the sense of validation I get from it. By validation, I mean the feeling that I am a successful, worthy human being – essentially, a sense of approval from others. It feels almost like a form of self-harm, because I know it's doing nothing but making me feel worse, but it's very difficult to stop.

Whereas as a child I was cutting myself with a maths compass to try and fit in with my friends who came into school with deep red scratches on their wrists, today I can log onto social media and invisibly rip myself apart. As in 'Z is for Zen', the rates of self-harm have skyrocketed in recent years, along with diagnosis of other mental health conditions, particularly in children. Deliberately engaging in activities that cause us harm, regardless of how visible it is, can fool us into feeling a false sense of control in an uncontrollable world. This choice simply keeps you stuck and unable to access any real control over your situation, because you're keeping yourself in it.

---

[41] Alex Reshanov, Getting fewer 'likes' on social media can make teens anxious and depressed : NewsCenter (rochester.edu), 24 September 2020. Accessed 17 March 2022: www.rochester.edu/newscenter/getting-fewer-likes-on-social-media-can-make-teens-anxious-and-depressed-453482/

Social media makes us all the stars of our own reality shows. We can open our profiles and see a highlights reel of our own lives, and notifications flood our brain with dopamine, overdosing us on the excitement of attention. It puts us on an endless upward battle of trying to feel 'enough' by external opinions of people we might not even know – we will never achieve it, no matter how many followers or likes we get. We simply cannot control how other people view us. In the meantime, we're driven to post more and more.

When I was chasing the most Instagrammable life around the world, I felt like my life was season 9 of a soap opera, where the writers had run out of storylines and were just mushing random decisions together that made no sense. I was obsessed with one-upping myself, and living the most outrageous and exciting life possible - or making it look like I was.

Social media puts us in the odd situation of being jealous of ourselves. Just like I compared the 'real' me to the model version of me in magazines as a teenager, we're all now able to compare our real lives to our virtual highlights reel. This feels like it should be achievable because we can literally see it on our screens, leading to us needing to keep up appearances by presenting a fake image of our lives to the world.

Narcissism

Narcissism is an associated with a personality disorder affecting 1% of the population, of an over-exaggerated sense of self-importance, a lack of empathy for others, a need for excessive admiration, and the belief that you are unique and deserving of special treatment. Essentially, being self-obsessed. As a coach, I've spoken to many women who worry they're narcissists. I tell them that narcissists don't worry about being narcissists!

However, social media can easily bring similar traits out in us, with tools design to over-stimulate the reward parts of our brains. Recognition is a natural thing to want, but most people simply don't have lives that are extreme enough to go viral on the internet every day. As a result, we can actively seek out opportunities to get more engagement online, which typically involves competing with ourselves to keep up appearances of how cool our lives are. Having done this myself for years, I know how empty and meaningless it makes these objectively amazing experiences. Just look at how many people take photographs of themselves in museums, instead of looking at the art!

When I was on the beach in Byron Bay, I couldn't enjoy it, because all I was doing was scrolling on my phone to see who cared that I was on the beach. I couldn't enjoy being on a photoshoot, because I was obsessively checking how many people had viewed my story. I couldn't enjoy going on holiday, because I was determined to get a perfect video of the hotel room before I touched anything inside it, and then spent *hours* editing it. I couldn't stop posting pictures of myself online, because I needed to feel like I was being seen.

What we think is narcissism today can often simply be an addiction to validation. It's a horrible way to live, where our sense of happiness is dependent on having something to post online, which wears off almost instantly. When we become dependent on validation, especially through platforms designed to exploit this vulnerability, it's obvious that we start thinking about it all the time.

Whenever I've gone through periods of having no social media, the strongest cravings to return have always been when I've gone on holiday. I noticed the compulsion to post a photo online of how cool my life was, as though I *wanted* other people to feel jealous of me – even though I don't want anyone to feel bad about themselves!

I noticed how much I beat myself up for not being able to understand why I wanted other people to feel jealous of me, or whether I just wished certain people were there with me. In this way, posting online could be more of a 'wish you were here' postcard, but social media blurs these lines.

Superiority & insecurity

When we live on our own reality tv shows, it's natural to feel competitive with other shows on the channel. Social media can distort how we see other people in this way, because it's easy to convince ourselves that people are jealous of *us*, which can make us feel threatened.

We're naturally and subconsciously judging other people online, which can influence how we post ourselves, as in 'J is for Jealousy'. The people we compare ourselves to highlight our insecurities.

This is especially important to remember when we think they're 'copying' us or want to be like us, because these odd feelings can turn into an annoying obsession, where we're competing with someone who might not even realise! It's like being forced to play a game of tennis by yourself – you realise how pointless it is but can't stop hitting the ball.

Measurements

The point of posting anything online is seeking validation, no matter how morally important our views are. We're saying that we matter, but this is distorted when we become dependent on the feedback to feel like this is true – it turns into us *asking* if we matter. I used to be unable to post a photo on Instagram without asking my friends first to choose which one and was always deleting them an hour later if they didn't get enough likes.

I was dependent on validation from the outside world to feel like I existed, but I could never get enough. I obsessed over the number of followers, likes, and comments I had to measure whether I was a worthy human being, trying everything I could to control them – but nothing worked. This had replaced the feeling I'd grown up with of only being worthy if I'd been booked on a modelling job. After having been unable to control this for years, having Instagram made me think I could somehow influence my career, if only I got enough followers. Instead of this, I just lost more and more control over my life.

This can happen in subtle ways, like provoking entire narratives of how unpopular we are after seeing a friend comment on another friend's post. These broken measurements give us an unreliable way of tracking our own self-worth, for example by allowing us to see if someone we're dating is following other people who could be considered attractive. Before we know it, we can easily lose hours of our lives to stalking people online that we'll probably never even meet!

Social media gives us the gambling machine version of validation – allowing us to pull a lever repeatedly in the hope of getting it right. It can fuel an obsession with fixing ourselves, as a misguided way of feeling like we can get some control over this game. As in 'S is for Surgery', this will never make us feel happy – we're always going to be looking for something else to fix. These games are simply impossible to win, but it's hard to step away if we don't even realise we're playing.

Guilt

When I posted modelling pictures online to appear 'booked and busy', I used to also feel as though I was making other people feel bad about themselves. I also felt both bad and good at the same time in 'one-upping' other models, imagining how they'd compare themselves to me as I did to them. This year, I've been modelling without having an Instagram account, and it's been bizarre to realise that I can simply turn up to work, do a job, and go home without having the extra hit of posting it online. It completely removes this guilty feeling, because I'm not expecting any reactions from other people about it.

Guilt underlies a lot of our need for validation. We're in the cycle of needing to keep up appearances around how wonderful our lives are going, feel bad for lying and compare ourselves to others, then post more to make ourselves feel better momentarily, before feeling guilty again for lying. Then we feel guilty for feeling guilty and spending so much time thinking about ourselves in this cycle!

It's easy to see this in an extreme way: we're either narcissistic for showing off or guilty for not showing off at all. Promoting and thinking about yourself isn't a bad thing – it's only if this leaves you feeling bad about yourself or other people. There's a brilliant woman called Stefanie Sword-Williams, who has a platform and book called Fuck Being Humble, who promotes self-promotion in a healthy way.

Social media gives us the opportunity to get so wrapped up in these extremes that we're yo-yoing between them in an ironically self-obsessed, but self-hating way. We can become addicted to 'fixing' ourselves and playing this out online. The aim is to find a middle, balanced ground that works for us.

Often, we can seek validation from the outside world as an attempt to fix how we feel on the inside, but we need to start with ourselves. We can start seeking validation from *ourselves* by treating ourselves as we would a small child in our care – listening to our own needs and desires each day, and consciously noticing the great things we do. Ultimately, the decision of whether you're 'enough' of anything is down to one person only: you. You are the only one who gets to truly decide that for yourself.

Tips

- How much time do you spend thinking about yourself? Is this usually in a positive or negative way?
- How worthy do you feel as a human being right now? How do you measure your self-worth?
- Try to write down what your pneeds are every day, and figure out how you can validate yourself. It can also be really helpful to write yourself a letter and literally give yourself the validation you're seeking!

- Identify an activity you could do to feel better in yourself, such as taking up music lessons. When we practice and develop a skill over time, our self-confidence improves.

- Think of a baby, who is loved for simply existing. Can you apply this same methodology to yourself? How can you recognise your own self-worth, regardless of anybody else's opinions?

- Can you identify one person who you can reach out to and share your successes with, encouraging them to do the same back?

- As you understand what makes you feel insecure and how you seek may seek validation unhealthily, can you take action to stop this from happening in the future? This might include switching off your 'likes' on social media, deleting apps from your home screen, or noticing when you start thinking insecurely about yourself and deciding to do something nice for yourself instead.

- The need for validation can come in waves and is often related to what's happening in our 'real' life, so if you notice this popping up, can you take a break from social media for a while? This would allow you to deal with the underlying issues, before returning.

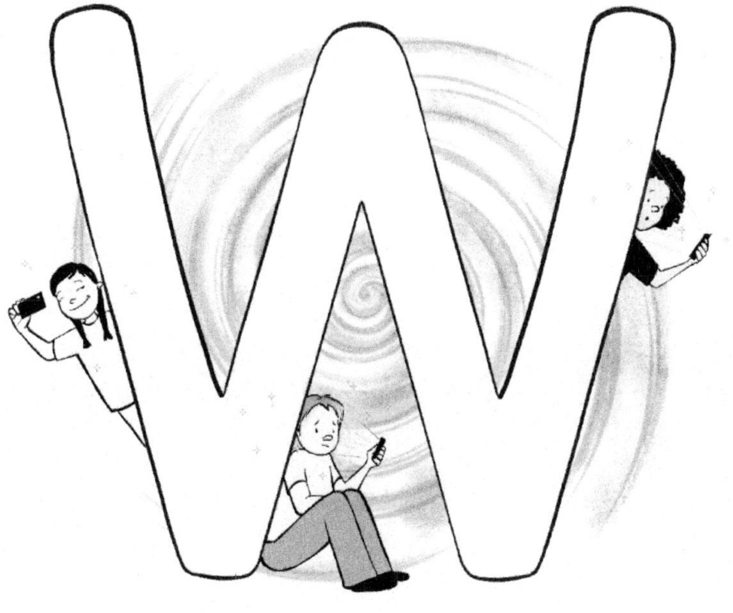

is for Weaknesses

W is for Weaknesses

Did you know?

- In 2013, ex-Google employee Tristan Harris made an internal presentation warning about human vulnerabilities that technology products were exploiting, abusing our natural psychological weaknesses to keep us addicted. This presentation, 'A Call to Minimize Distraction and Respect Users' Attention', went viral.[42]

Human beings all share the same inherent aspects and core needs, which in some situations, can be used in certain ways to influence us, such as by magicians, or advertisers. As we're not given a guidebook of being human upon birth, it's natural to blame ourselves when we fall into a scrolling vortex, for example, without realising that our human vulnerabilities are being exploited.

We're not robots or algorithms – we have emotions and biases programmed into us that can overcome our willpower in certain situations. This explains things like procrastination, distraction, mistakes and essentially any situation where our behaviour doesn't match what we want. It can be very frustrating to feel out of control of your own mind and body, but beating yourself up for this only reinforces the cycle: it's not your fault.

When I was addicted to Instagram and dating apps, I asked everyone I knew how to stop self-sabotaging. They all told me the same thing: willpower. 'You just do it', they said. This is an incredibly frustrating thing to be told when you *know* what you need to do, but seem to be

---

[42] Casey Newton, 'Google's new focus on well-being started five years ago with this presentation' - The Verge, 10 May 2018. Accessed 17 March 2022.

incapable of actually doing it. The willpower button seemed to not be working in my brain, which made it feel like someone else had the remote control to my life. It was only by learning about my brain, to understand these vulnerabilities and 'weaknesses', that I could put strategies in place to protect them from exploitation by others and start being in control of my own life.

The below human traits are weaknesses only because they are inherent evolutionary vulnerabilities in all of us that are being exploited by social media. Once we understand them, we can remind ourselves that we're not living in the same world our ancestors were, and take control over our own decisions.

1. Bad predictions – especially with time!

Have you ever fallen down a scrolling vortex, not realising that you've spent far longer than you intended on your phone? As in 'T is for Time', there's a reason that social media companies email us tantalizing updates such as 'you've been tagged in a photo', or 'someone has sent you a message', or send us signals to this effect, instead of simply telling us what we need to know. These alerts excite the dopamine in our brain, just like a present under the Christmas tree waiting to be unwrapped.

Ultimately, the point is to get us to log in and get distracted. When our attention is held by the continuous novelty rollercoaster of a social media feed, we can easily lose track of time. Research has shown that it takes us over 23 minutes to get back to what we were doing when we get distracted! When we were all living in caves, our brains were designed to focus primarily on the present moment rather than planning for the future, because surviving was much harder!

It's easy to convince ourselves that we're in control of this, especially if we've had the experience of losing track of time on our phones before. However, when we enter into the social media vortex, it's us vs the world's most intelligent behavioural design engineers, who have studied how to keep us trapped every time. Despite telling ourselves that we'll watch 'just one more' video, our brain is being tricked into forgetting this and staying plugged in.

Solution: turn notifications off, and unsubscribe from email updates from social media apps. We do not need to be drip-fed these updates throughout the day, but can easily check them all in one go, when *we* want to, instead of when we're being manipulated. To do this, we have to recognise that we are simply can't win against the people setting these notifications alone, which is strangely liberating!

2. **Intermittent Variable Rewards – aka the excitement of uncertainty and novelty**

Our neurotransmitter of dopamine gets excited by uncertainty and novelty, because it keeps us striving to achieve new things. If our ancestors became too used to one kind of crop, for example, and ate it all, our species wouldn't have survived to the next generation, so this is what keeps us motivated to grow and seek out new experiences.

In the same way, humans typically feel a lot more 'lust' in the first few weeks of a new relationship with somebody than 10 years in, because we're evolutionally motivated to find a partner and continue our species. As in 'L is for Love', dating apps are extremely addictive in this way because we can't predict how things will play out when we finally meet the person we've built up a story about in our minds. We get the same high every time we check our emails, text messages, or notifications, because it's all about anticipating what's happened since we last checked.

As in 'A is for Algorithms', algorithms on social media are designed to show us whatever will be the most 'engaging' content when we log in, constantly stimulating this novelty-seeking part of our brain. When Instagram's algorithm was chronological, we might have been dependent on the people we followed to post new content to see new things, which meant we could log out after reading new updates since our last log in. However, now we can continuously refresh the page to keep getting the high of stimulation.

TikTok is particularly dangerous for this, because its algorithms promote content seemingly at random, regardless of how many followers a person has. Completely unpredictable algorithms such as this, which hold what may seem like potentially huge 'rewards' of going viral overnight, can lead people to obsessively keep trying in the hope of 'winning'. As in 'X is for X-rated', this can also lead to posting sexually suggestive content to try and figure out the algorithm.

Solution: when we understand how social media keeps us hooked, just like we're playing a slot machine in a casino, we can decide to use this only with serious conscious control. For example, deleting the apps from your phone and only going on them on a desktop computer will remove the addictive 'swiping' to refresh feature, so I'd advise making it as difficult as you can to get onto the apps and only using them when you really want to, with a pre-defined purpose.

3. Fear of missing out

1000 years ago, if we weren't popular with our peers, we might have been at risk of being left behind and dying. If we didn't stay in the know of where the pack was moving to next, or what dangers lay ahead, we could have faced genuine life or death situations.

This explains our instinctual human desire to stay 'in the know' and to be liked by other people – apart from the obvious fact that having strong human connections is crucial for our survival. Social media amplifies the school-ground fear of not being invited to the cool kid's birthday party by a billion per cent – we can simply never keep up to date with everything that happens online!

At the same time, we're also given torturous windows into people's lives that make us feel like we're losing out by not having what they have, as in 'J is for Jealousy'. The hundreds of notifications we get every day can condition us to believe that we 'need' to check our phones throughout the day in case of a situation happening where we somehow lose our social status as a result. Our brain can process this as a genuine life or death situation, as an attempt to feel in control of the uncontrollable. Ironically, this is keeping us in a state of constant panic and fear, instead of stability – checking our phones 'just in case' becomes a safety behaviour that we depend on to feel secure.

Solution: deliberately 'miss out'. When we don't know what is happening, we don't care about it – simple! We stop worrying about the parties or meet ups we're not invited to, because we don't have to watch them playing out on social media. As in 'R is for Resilience', doing this also proves to us that there is more to life than this virtual world. By having days off certain apps or the internet all together, you can help condition your brain to feel secure in reality, rather than worrying about what you're missing. If something happens that you really need to know about, someone will tell you – trust me!

4. Subconscious decisions

Have you ever travelled somewhere, and forgotten how you ended up there? Our brains have to make thousands of decisions each day, and if these were all conscious, we'd probably explode! When we make a conscious decision, such as what to cook for dinner, this is a very different process to one that's subconscious, such as eating chocolate from a box in front of you whilst doing something else.

This is because of how much effort we put into the thinking process – when we pause and consider something, this takes up more brain energy, and involves us making a deliberate action. When we act mindlessly, this is usually more of an immediate reaction to our environment, removing the ability for us to stop and think.

Social media exploits this by making the 'user experience' as seamless and frictionless as possible. When the decision is made for us, such as a new video automatically playing on Youtube or Netflix, or endless scrolling on Instagram, it can be very mentally difficult to fight back against this. It requires more brain energy in considering whether this is what we want to do. As in 'M is for Money', this is easily exploited by apps making it possible to pay for things with the press of a button, instead of physically having to use our cards or cash.

Apps like TikTok are incredibly addictive because it is making these subconscious choices for us so quickly that we barely have time to make a decision before we're being shown the next video, which has been tailored uniquely to our individual interests. In China, the Government requires the equivalent app to have a 5 second break between videos for children, with notifications urging them to get off their phones – and TikTok is a Chinese app!

Solution: set up 'speed bumps' for all of the things you want to think about more, such as uninstalling your bank cards from your phone, or deleting apps from your home screen. The more friction you can set for yourself in the online world, the more time you'll have to make your own decisions!

5. Stress

Social media can cause such an overload of stimulation that our sympathetic nervous system is activated, preparing to go into 'fight or flight mode'. When our ancestors encountered a bear hundreds of years ago, adrenaline would surge throughout their body, increasing their heart rate in preparation for fighting or running away as quickly as possible. They wouldn't have been in the best place to make decisions about what to eat for dinner at that point!

Today, every time we go on our phones we can enter similar physiological states. For example, we could easily be 'cancelled' for things we didn't know were wrong, or receive abuse online, as in 'K is for Kindness'. We can be shown scary news updates which may not even be true, as in 'U is for Unreal', and traumatic content. We have no idea what awaits us, every time we log on to our innocent looking social media apps.

If we check our phones 100-300 times per day, this is keeping us locked into a permanent state of worry and stress. This makes it very difficult to make good decisions, because our ability to think rationally is impacted by a constant state of anxiety. Frustratingly, we may have no idea this is even happening, as we keep returning to social media in an attempt to 'relax'.

Solution: de-stress yourself. By only checking your messages and apps at certain times of the day, for limited periods, you can confine the amount of exposure you have to these stressful situations. It's also good to ensure you relax each day in ways that that aren't related to technology, such as going for a walk or doing yoga.

6. Negativity bias

As in 'C is for Content', humans have a bias to automatically focus more on negativity than positivity. Our ancestors had to be more aware of potential dangers than they were of what was already going well, because they were under constant threats to their survival. We hardly have any of those same threats (such as being eaten by predators!), but we've still got this inbuilt tendency to worry and focus on what could go wrong, instead of what could go right.

This human vulnerability can be exploited on social media to show us more and more extreme, scary situations, that keep us locked in anxious states, which can filter out into the rest of our lives, making us believe things are worse than they actually are.

Solution: focus on the positives! When we know we have a bias towards negativity, can you notice every negative thought and balance it out with a positive one? The 'worst case scenario' is just as likely to happen as the 'best case scenario'. Gratitude journaling is also extremely helpful to remind yourself regularly of all the positives around you.

7. Us vs them

As we evolved in tribes of people, we can easily categorise people into groups that are either 'like us' or 'not like us'. Humans have a 'confirmation bias', which means we look for information that confirms what we already believe. When our beliefs aren't being challenged, because we simply avoid exposure to anything different, it's easy for us to see people with different beliefs as 'bad', just because they don't think like us on certain issues.

We also have a tendency to follow the crowd, also knowing as 'anchoring', which is when we look to other people to shape our beliefs. This is often seen with comments under news articles, for example, when the top rated comments are all similar to each other. It can feel safer to be a sheep and follow 'groupthink', but this can become very problematic when we stop connecting with our own beliefs. This can easily lead us into extremist thoughts, without us realising quite how we'd reached that point.

As in 'K is for Kindness', people are not either all 'good' or all 'bad'. Just imagine if we believed everybody that didn't share our religious belief were inherently 'bad', for example!

Solution: try to seek out different points of views to yours, and to understand them. Try to read news from a different political standpoint to yours, and think through the arguments in a logical way. If you have beliefs you're especially passionate about, try to put yourself in the shoes of someone who doesn't share these. Can you still find empathy for them, and think of a way you could explain your point of view in a calm and logical way? Why do you believe what you believe?

8. Social comparisons based on our appearance

Just as we've always had to fight for popularity to evolve as human beings, we've had to compete with other people. Interestingly, females have evolved to be more visually focused, which is why apps like Instagram may impact girls and women so negatively. In the days of hunter-gatherers, men would typically be out hunting animals, and women would be more focused on gathering plants to eat. Men would've adapted to adrenaline-based 'wins' (much like video-games today), and women would've adapted to noticing subtle visual differences.

Women would also have been more focused on appealing to men to bear their children, as monogamy is a relatively new concept for us! It was very normal for men to have children with lots of different women. These evolutionary instincts help explain our society's obsession with appearances today, as in 'B is for Beauty'. Women especially, are hard-wired to focus on appearances – and the difference between being 'beautiful' or not, could have meant the difference between life and death.

Over one-third of our brains are dedicated to processing visual information, which helps explain why apps focusing on visual content are so successful. Ones that literally place visual content alongside each other makes it virtually impossible not to compare the posts, especially if it relates to us personally, which is why apps such as Instagram can be so damaging for our self-esteem.

Solution: avoid environments which allow you to compare yourself. This may mean limiting the amount of time you spend on apps such as Instagram, and being very conscious of when you start to feel insecure about how you look. Be pro-active in consciously complimenting yourself each day, and remember how uniquely perfect you are, exactly as you are.

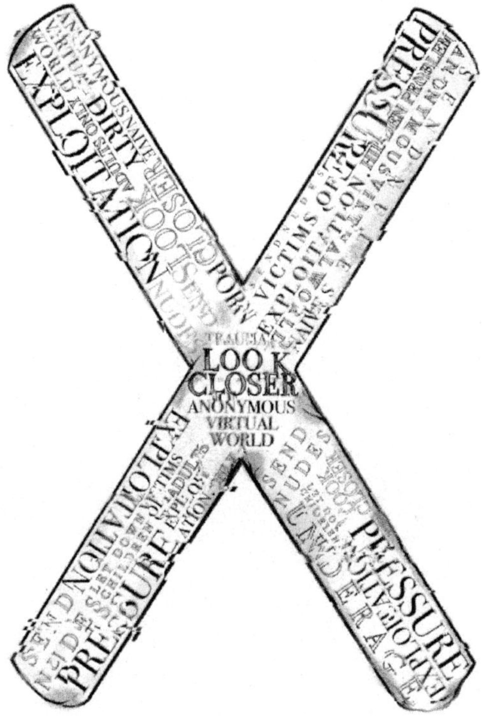

is for X-rated

X is for X-rated

Did you know?

- Children as young as 7 or 8 years old are watching online pornography. A study found around 53% of 11-16 year olds had seen explicit material online, nearly all of whom (94%) had seen it by age 14. Research by the British Board of Film Classification found teenagers are increasingly using explicit content as a way of learning about sex.[43]

As a child, stylists would instruct me how to pose on photoshoots for magazines. Right from my very first shoot which appeared in *Vogue*, I was positioned in ways that made me feel uncomfortable, but I couldn't figure out why. I was told to look 'sexy', to grab my crotch, to put a hand inside my bra, suck my fingers, and to lean inside car windows, arch my back and 'stick my bum out'.

There are photos of me as a child which make me feel incredibly uncomfortable to look at, because it's only by growing older, that I understand how sexualised I was – and mostly for women's fashion magazines! Sex is everywhere in our society, but it's still highly repressed and difficult to speak about in an open and clear way.

I was first introduced to sex by a pop-up advert on the home computer, of naked adults doing things that I couldn't understand. I remember being horrified by puberty hitting my body, and trying to figure out whether I was a 'freak' by asking other girls in my class. It simply wasn't spoken about at home. I don't remember ever receiving any kind of sex education in school, except from boys who

---

[43] Siobhan Smith, 'How to talk about porn with your children and teenagers' | Metro News, 9 March 2022. Accessed 17 March 2022.

asked me to give them 'blow jobs', and me trying to figure out what on earth this meant.

Whereas I and probably most of my generation figured this out by talking to each other, if we were growing up today, we would've been able to use the internet. As in 'A is for Algorithms', if I'd googled 'blow job', I would quickly have been led down a rabbit hole of hard-core pornography.

Porn

Today, the largest group of internet porn consumers is children aged between 12-17.[44] Porn websites feature heavily in the top 10 websites of the world: it's pointless trying to pretend it doesn't exist to children, who are probably more technologically advanced than most adults. Despite this obvious reality, and sex alluded to almost everywhere in our society, there is still a huge sense of stigma and shame about speaking about sex. Sex education in school focuses largely on biology and dangers of getting pregnant, often completely missing out large topics such as masturbation or different kinds of sexual activity. Unsurprisingly, the gaps lead to children looking for the answers online.

Singer Billie Eilish explained how as an 11-year-old watching porn, she thought this was how people 'learned how to have sex'. She explained how it destroyed her brain, gave her nightmares, and caused her to find it hard to say no to sexual experiences, because she 'thought that was what [she] was supposed to be attracted to'.[45]

When children are learning how to have sex from the internet, they think this is 'normal'. Videos of women apparently enjoying being degraded gives signals to those watching that this is what they like.

---

[44] 'Internet Statistics', *GuardChild*, accessed 20 February 2022. www.guardchild.com/statistics/

[45] 'Billie Eilish says porn exposure while young caused nightmares', *BBC News*, 14 December 2021. Accessed 20 February 2022. www.bbc.co.uk/news/entertainment-arts-59658663

However, the internet Is not an educational resource free of bias or other influences. The same algorithms that keep people hooked on social media platforms apply to the world of porn: they want to keep the user 'engaged'.

Watching 'ordinary' sex of the kind found in average human encounters might create a dopamine spike of doing something 'naughty' the first time it's viewed by someone. Then, it will become normal. To get the same spike, a viewer might click on the next video in line, which might feature something more violent or shocking. It continues in this way until the viewer has become completely numb to 'normal' human sexual experiences, and needs the high of watching something they find disgusting to be able to reach the same point – just like a drug.

Our brains can't tell the difference between a naked person standing in front of us, and a photo of them. So, it's natural that we seek out human interactions by watching porn to feel the illusion of a hit of a sexual connection, when in reality, there's only one person involved. This false version of connection simply leaves us feeling even more lonely than before. The intimate, yet often violent, nature of online pornography can also leave us feeling shameful and disgusted with ourselves, as in 'K is for Kindness'.

Porn can easily turn 'real life' sex into something that is less stimulating than its online alternative, especially when considering the messy human emotions and awkwardness involved, as in 'R is for Resilience'. However, just like having a heroin addiction might feel good for the addict when high, but bad the rest of the time, there's a reason that being addicted to porn is a serious problem.

I've known men who have been unable to orgasm in real life due to watching porn. This is because their brains have literally changed in response to the material they've been watching, and real human interactions can't ever meet the same highs. It's like taking paracetamol after taking cocaine every day: they may hardly even feel it. This is in a similar way to how our brains can adapt to filtered content online, making it difficult to enjoy the mundanity of 'real life' in comparison, as in 'U is for Unreal'.

Violence

When our brains believe sex, or real life in general, should imitate porn, there's a serious risk of harm to the people involved. In 2021, a website called 'Everyone's Invited' exploded with tens of thousands of women and girls' testimonies about a normalised culture of misogyny, molestation and sexual harassment whilst growing up in the UK. The #MeToo movement demonstrated how global sexual harassment of women has been simply normalised and accepted for decades.

Porn doesn't typically display consent, boundaries, or genuine connection. It tends to be hyper-sexualised, graphic, violent, and generally, unrealistic. If I'd ended up googling the sexual requests made of me as a teenager, I probably would have thought these were completely normal, and my uncomfortableness was me being 'frigid'. It wasn't until I spoke to an older woman about some experiences that I was having in an abusive relationship that I understood these weren't normal – if we don't have any reference points, how are we supposed to know?

This normalization of violence against women is seen on social media, where it's normal for public figures such as female members of Parliament or influencers to receive detailed rape and death threats. As in 'K is for Kindness', receiving this kind of abuse has simply become normalised online, which is reflected throughout our society.

Nudity

This over-exposure to graphic content is mirrored in social media today. Apps such as Snapchat and Whatsapp allow users to send 'disappearing messages', which can give the illusion of safety in sending someone an explicit photograph. I've head of Snapchat groups where every girl is expected to contribute with a nude picture of themselves, or to be deemed uncool.

50% of surveyed children aged between 9 and 17 reported sending nude photographs to a person they'd never met in real life, with 41% of respondents believing they were sending the images to an adult.[46] Being sent unsolicited graphic images of sexual content has become normal, from simply being 'airdropped' a photo on the train from a stranger, to them sliding into direct messages on social media. This is despite the fact that looking at or having content featuring children is a criminal offence.

Having disappearing messages doesn't mean that content disappears – once it's sent, it can be on the internet forever. This can be easily used as pressure to send content you're uncomfortable with, as though refusing to do so implies that you'd think the person would screenshot it, or don't trust them!

As in 'R is for Resilience', it's unsurprising that many people today feel in a state of constant anxiety, with the possibility of people we trust betraying us by having such a huge amount of power over us. Today, there's even the possibility of 'deep fakes', with altered images to put anybody's face into a pornographic context, as in 'U is for Unreal'!

As everybody today has a smartphone, there's the potential to be photographed or filmed by virtually anyone we're in intimate situations with. As a model being sent to photographer's houses for photoshoots, I've become automatically untrusting of any new scenario where I'm expected to get undressed, always checking for potential cameras, knowing other models who have been filmed changing. This danger is easy to forget when it's so normalised to

---

[46] 'Thorn research: Trends confirm need for parents to talk about online safety with kids earlier, more often', *Thorn,* 12 November 2021. Accessed 20 February 2022. www.thorn.org/blog/thorn-research-trends-confirm-need-for-parents-to-talk-about-online-safety-with-kids-earlier-more-often/

meet strangers from the internet and potentially end up at their house because we feel like we know them, as in 'L is for Love'.

Sexualisation

As we've all become both content and content creators, social media has allowed for an avalanche of sexual 'empowerment'. Even though we might take a sexual photo of ourselves and feel good about this, as soon as we post it online, there's the expectation of a reaction, as in 'V is for Validation'.

Social media has both normalised and manipulated this, as algorithms tend to promote this type of sexualised, 'shocking' content, because human beings are simply biologically drawn to sexual images. This can result in situations of 'influencers' having large followings that are mostly made up of people who are sexually attracted to them, instead of an audience that cares about what they think. It can also see people who want to get more followers posting more sexualised content of themselves, as they think this is what will be more likely to get likes.

There are also platforms such as OnlyFans, which give an illusion of 'sexual empowerment' by people being able to post what is often graphic content of themselves in return for money. When our society puts people on pedestals for literally having their sex tapes released publicly, this can very incorrectly link sexualised content to fame and 'success'. Model Emily Ratajowski spoke about how she previously labelled her involvement in the 'Blurred Lines' music video as empowering, despite being sexual harassed during the shoot.

Sexual 'empowerment' through social media in this way can often be a frustrating attempt to get control over our own bodies, because ultimately, the people in power remain the same. As a model, regardless of whether I'm being pressured to pose naked by a photographer or am posting these images myself in return for payment, ultimately, other people are benefiting from the objectification of my body, as in 'O is for Objectification'. This can lead us to see our bodies as separate tools to get things we want, instead of as part of who we are. When we are 'rewarded' for our sexuality on the internet, we can easily come to believe that our value is in how we look, and base our self-esteem on this.

Saying no

I've also been pressured to get undressed by photographers throughout my modelling career, understanding how subtle manipulations can make us feel guilty and awkward for saying no. I was fortunate that this was in a supposedly 'professional' context and I felt like I had a 'reason' for saying no, in wanting to become a lawyer later on, but many other people don't have this 'reason'.

This is extremely difficult when people around us are acting as though we're being unreasonable. I once had a horrible shoot for a magazine where the female photographer was pressuring me to spank another model with a ping pong bat and pose as though we were having sex. I was crying, and she instructed me to just 'hide my face with my hair'. This is the world that so many people are in today – where they're being made to feel unreasonable for not wanting to do something that makes them feel uncomfortable.

Ultimately, there is a lot of stigma and shame attached to sex in our society, but it doesn't have to be like this. By speaking about it and seeking support from others, the shame is instantly reduced. Having sexual feelings is not shameful – you are a completely normal and acceptable human being.

Even if you've somehow ended up watching very bizarre things on the internet that don't make you feel good about yourself, this doesn't mean you are necessarily attracted to or even agree with those things. If there's content of you online that you feel uncomfortable with, don't worry about it, but simply move on with your life and decide to implement your boundaries going forward. There's no point in worrying about the things we can't control, but we CAN control our own bodies and boundaries in the future. Every experience serves as a valuable lesson for next time!

Tips

- Assess what your relationship is with sex and boundaries. How confident do you feel with your sexual identity, and saying no to situations you're uncomfortable with?
- Does pornography or sexualised content feature in your life at all? What's the impact of this on you? How do you feel about this in comparison to 'real' sex? Can you tell the difference between this and what real sex should be like?
- Try to communicate what you are and are not comfortable with. For example, saying, 'I'm not comfortable with that', is a full sentence – as is 'no'. Can you identify situations where you could be compromised in setting these boundaries, such as those involving alcohol? How can you stay safe in these situations and ensure you are respected?
- How do you want to feel about content featuring you online? You don't need to have a reason to not post or create things like this. For example, I have always had a very strong boundary of simply never sending photos I'm not comfortable with. If the other person has an issue with this, it's their issue – not mine. They could be the nicest, most trustworthy person in the world, but phones are still vulnerable to being hacked. This decision should only involve one person: you.
- Try not to share any content you feel uncomfortable with. If someone is pressuring you do to so, this is a red flag about their intentions towards you, and I'd strongly recommend speaking support from someone you trust.

- If you watch pornography or view highly sexualised content, does this make you feel good on balance, or does it impact your day-to-day relationships in some way? If so, can you consider limiting your exposure to these things and focusing on the 'real' relationships? Your brain will very quickly adapt to enjoying real life more than the concentrated version of it, but for some people, porn can essentially be an addiction that you need to wean yourself off to be able to fully enjoy sexual experiences without it.

- Try going to life drawing classes, to see nudity in a non-sexualised context.

- Find someone you trust to speak with about these issues, such as a therapist.

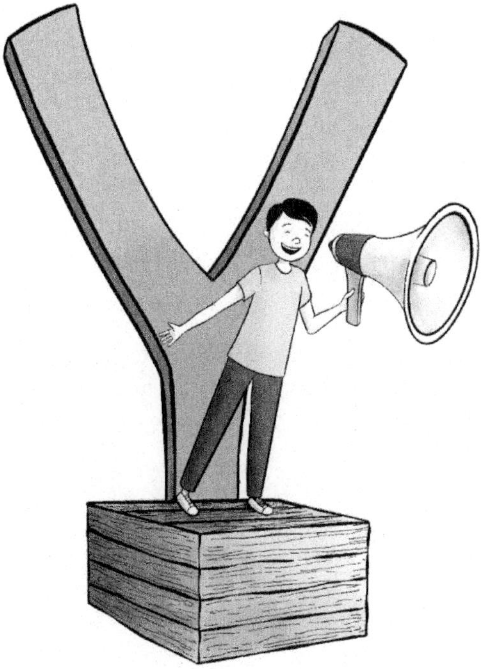

is for Your Truth

Y is for Your truth

Did you know?

- 61% of millennials get their news primarily through social media. We tend to engage most with information that flatters our ideological preconceptions, which relates most to selection bias, than algorithmic filtering: we like to see things that confirm what we already believe.[47]

By the time I was diagnosed with ADHD age 25, I'd self-diagnosed myself with at least 5 different conditions, none of which were ADHD, and none of which I had. However, once I'd turned to Google to figure out why I wasn't happy 100% of the time, I couldn't stop, until I'd paid £400 for an appointment with a private psychiatrist. The possibilties are endless, and all extremely relatable, as in 'C is for Content'.

I spoke to someone recently who'd resonated with an article she'd read about ADHD in the news and been diagnosed within 24 hours on zoom, paying thousands of pounds. There is no physical test that can be done to confirm this diagnosis – it's simply going based on a series of standardised, arguably outdated questions, and usually some feedback by other people in your life describing how you were as a child.

This can all happen so quickly that it can leave you questioning how it could be possible for someone to change your life and identity so dramatically within a few minutes, especially if they're profiting significantly from this. I couldn't believe I was expected to pay £300

---

[47] David Robert Grimes, 'Echo chambers are dangerous – we must try to break free of our online bubbles' | The Guardian, 4 December 2017. Accessed 17 March 2022.

per month to a private psychiatrist for *the rest of my life* to take medication I apparently needed for my mental health that would be too difficult to access on the NHS. When people around me were saying ADHD was something made up to exploit vulnerable people, I was more inclined to believe them because of this, even though I knew something was seriously wrong.

Once you're diagnosed, no one gives you guidance on what this means, or how the medication you might have been prescribed should make you feel, and so you search for the answers online. There's a limitless world of information, communities, posts, videos, webinars, workshops and more for virtually every single niche subject we can think of. I wrote *ADHD: an A to Z* to help me collate and understand this information for myself.

The problem with having this world of information at our fingertips, is that we can't process it properly. It becomes extremely difficult to tell what's real or fake, what's an advertisement or sale, what's right or wrong – including our own thoughts, beliefs and values. If we don't realise these are up for sale to the highest bidder, we're at risk of being manipulated to the point of ultimately being unable able to trust ourselves.

Fake news

20 years ago, most people got their news from newspapers, which were printed once a day. Today, almost half of UK adults use social media for news.[48] As in 'C is for Content', it's much more likely that the news we see will be negative than positive, because the intention is to make us stay on the page, as we are exposed to paid advertising. As in 'R is for Resilience', being exposed to negative content in this way can easily make us feel as though things are much worse than

---

[48] 'News Consumption in the UK: 2021', *Ofcom*, 27 July 2021. Accessed 20 February 2022.
www.ofcom.org.uk/__data/assets/pdf_file/0025/222478/news-consumption-in-the-uk-overview-of-findings-2021.pdf

they are in reality. For example, news coverage of the 9/11 hijacking of a plane by terrorists resulted in a huge increase of Americans driving instead of flying, which was not only much more statistically dangerous, but also led to more road accidents happening due to an increase in traffic.

Terrorism has been likened to a 'fly in a china shop', because although the number of people killed in such attacks are generally very low in contrast to how many people there are in the world, it can be reported on so dramatically that we can feel as though it's a very real and constant danger. For example, I developed very frustrating habits of worrying about a potential attack every time I went on a train, which led to me changing train about 5 times each jouney I took! This quickly morphed into other obsessive compulsive type 'rules', like having to compliment a stranger in order to somehow have a safer journey.

I thought making up and following these rules helped me have some kind of control over the situation, but all it did was give me more complex versions of anxiety! Realistically, any of us could drop dead at any point for any reason, so what's the point in ruining our lives over trying to control this?

Checking the news can also be very addictive, especially in relation to seeking out novelty – we are conditioned to seeing 'new' news multiple times a day. Refreshing our Twitter feed to find out the latest update about a tense political situation on the other side of the world might feel like we're staying in control, but it's putting our brains under repeated stress, despite our believing that this might be 'soothing' our worries.

Whilst news publications are generally regulated, and have obligations to provide 'real' information, social media channels operate in a world of their own. Anybody can post a 'news' update, as seen during the Covid-19 pandemic, where at the time of writing, 6 million people in the UK are in conspiracy groups on Facebook. Huge political earthquakes like the Brexit referendum and Trump election demonstrate the potential for people's behaviour to be manipulated by news articles containing fake information.

This is often because lies are more exciting than the truth. We are simply more likely to click on an article about a missing child who has been found after a dramatic kidnap and police shoot-out, rather than one who simply ran away. As in 'A is for Algorithms', the over-supply of information can lead us to click on the most dramatic and easy to read posts, which can simplify complex issues into what we think is the 'truth'.

Echo chambers

What I see on a social media platform like Facebook might be completely different to what you see, even if we have identical lists of friends – we are literally being given different versions of virtual reality. This is because algorithms understand our different interests, and show us whatever is most likely to keep us on the platform. A large part of this may be showing us posts that confirm what we already believe, as we like to be validated. Different people are also likely to follow their own individual interests in the same way, which can lead to us existing in 'echo chambers'.

As in 'K is for Kindness', this can create serious difficulties when our beliefs about the world are formed from these platforms. If we're in a room of 1000 people who all disagree with our opinion, we're more likely to believe we might be mistaken. However, if they all agree with us, then we're more likely to believe the 1 person who has a different view is mistaken. Social media can make these invisible worlds real, because our beliefs are confirmed on a continuous basis to us through the day.

Although we can find people online who share our opinions, this can be more difficult in real life. We have to live and work alongside people whose views we may not agree with, but this doesn't necessarily make them terrible people – humans are very complex.

However, this can easily be forgotten on social media, with bitesize content, such as 180 character Tweets leading to drastic misunderstandings.

It's very challenging to talk about 'right' and 'wrong' opinions without knowing the full story. People are generally not 'good' or 'evil' – we've all had our own experiences which have led to why we believe what we do. However, if we typecast people into these binary categories, we can easily cause stress and conflict that doesn't need to exist. If contrary opinions to ours are refused to exist at all, then we can become more deeply buried into our echo chamber, are more likely to end up with extremist views, and may struggle to communicate with other people.

What's more, we can easily end up being exploited online by people who can easily predict our behaviour if we have such strong views. From buying products we don't need, to believing we need to change our bodies in some way, if our feelings are predictable, they are vulnerable to manipulation. Our insecurities are worth billions.

Our own truth

In contrast to setting the standards of what is 'true', social media also gives us the ability to set these ourselves. When Meghan Markle spoke out about the mental health struggles she'd experienced to Oprah, the world seemed divided on whether this 'really' happened or not. Regardless of whether it did, it was what she felt, so it seemed bizarre that everybody cared so much to the point of one television presenter leaving his job.

However, this is what happens when we set binary 'yes' or 'no' rules for public views – the internet has become a version of a court of law, and we've all been appointed as the jury. When we're all able to give our own version of reality and moral standards, this can create a highly anxious environment for us all in not knowing what the 'right' thing to say is. Instead of saying anything at all, many of us may simply stay silent out of fear of getting into conflict, with resentment slowly building up.

It's great that social media gives everybody the opportunity to use their voice and share their experiences, but we must remember to listen to others and be vulnerable to getting things wrong, without being shamed for this. No one can truly know what it's like to be anybody else, so we're all simply doing our best to co-operate in this gigantic world of human beings. Your perspective is extremely important, and so is everybody else's – but social media can trick us into thinking otherwise.

Our thoughts are not reality

The most valuable lesson I've learned in life is 'don't believe everything you think'. I didn't previously realise how much my brain was making up narratives about everything in my life, including myself. For example, I'd assume that if I didn't get a modelling job, this must be because I wasn't thin enough, due to being pressured to lose weight for many years – when this was probably not true at all! Even so, I would still beat myself up for this and crash diet.

Social media can give us the 'proof' for what we believe. As in 'F is for Friendships', I was constantly creating stories for why friends of mine hadn't liked my posts, or investigating whether they were possibly hanging out without me. We can easily take a person's online activity out of context as proof they don't really like us, or as though they are doing something wrong, such as following certain people.

Thinking like this is generally not useful – we often just end up frustrated at ourselves, as it's pretty awkward to tell someone you're annoyed with them because they haven't liked your posts! Instead of this, we might post more provocative content in the hope of getting a reaction, but we can't control other people – and especially not what they do online.

Tips

- Assess your beliefs: what are your morals, values and beliefs?
- Where do you get most of your news from? Do you agree with all of the articles? Can you imagine writing one from the opposite point of view?
- Look at different versions of the truth by reading the opposite political viewpoints on the same news. AllSides.com is a website showing balanced updates with all of the different poltitical takes on news stories, noting that studies show those who diversify their news consumption experience less anxiety around current events.
- If there's someone you strongly disagree with, can you try to speak to them about it in a calm way? If this isn't an option, can you try to put yourself in their shoes? Can you feel empathy for them and try to identify what may have led them to have the beliefs they have?
- Ultimately, people can believe whatever they want to, and all we can do is respect their right to do this. They are extremely unlikely to change their view on something, no matter how many fights you get into, but is this a reason to cut people out of your life who diasgree with you? Can you find a compromise on this and separate the person from their view?
- Remember that being so passionate about a viewpoint that we might be getting into fights with people about it is generally only going to keep us stuck in an angry stress cycle, and this energy could be much more productively used.
- Challenge your thoughts. When you're feeling annoyed or frustrated, try this exercise:

a) What is the thought that's bothering you? *(e.g X is a bad person because they have this view)*

b) Can you prove this to be 100% true? What evidence do you have? *(e.g X posted a status about their view)*

c) What is believing this thought doing to you? How do you act and think when you have this thought? Is it useful? *(e.g I got annoyed, got into an argument with X on their status, now keep getting more angry, and it's not useful.)*

d) What is the opposite belief? What proof do you have for this? *(e.g X is not a bad person. The proof I have for this is that they are usually nice to me and other people.)*

This simple exercise puts you in control of the sitaution, by allowing you to choose your thoughts, instead of reacting to them automatically. When it comes to truth, taking a step back from the internet can help us put things into perspective.

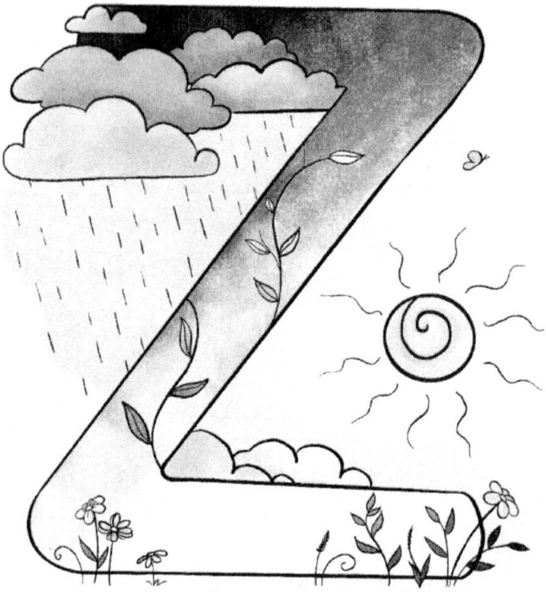

is for Zen

Z is for Zen

- Extremely high rates of depression, anxiety and self-harm in teenagers have been linked to heavy social media use, with a 40-year highs in suicide amongst teen girls. Even if this isn't the root cause, it's been referred to as possibly being 'an accelerant — the gasoline that turns a flicker of adolescent angst into a blaze.'[49]

Whilst the online world can be an excellent way of distracting ourselves from our feelings, it doesn't get rid of them. They bubble away subconsciously, still impacting how we feel about ourselves. Our repeated failed attempts to get control over our feelings, experiences, self-worth, popularity, appearance, and lives through social media can leave us feeling worse off, beating ourselves up for things that are simply not out fault.

For example, when making a short video for an app like TikTok, I can literally spend *hours* trying to match up words and songs and perfect execution, where all I'm concentrating on is the video. However, once I've posted the video and logged off, I feel a tidal wave of anxiety at how the post will do, anger and guilt at myself for wasting such a huge chunk of my time on something that I know is ultimately quite pointless, and worried about all the other things I have to do.

I might log back on to reassure myself by checking how the video is doing, and get sucked into a numbing scrolling vortex, as in 'T is for Time', losing even more of my day. This time when I log out, I might be beating myself up for not being as good the other videos I've

---

[49] Markham Heid, 'We Need to Talk About Kids and Smartphones' | Time, 10 October 2017. Accessed 17 March 2022.

subconsciously compared myself to. This can often end up with me logging back in to delete my original post!

Ultimately, our interaction with social media can sometimes be a way of self-harming ourselves without even realising. As technology develops, we might be able to invert ourselves more deeply into this online world, but we will always stay human beings – the body and mind come together as a package deal!

This means we're still going to have feelings, emotions, and human needs like sleeping, eating, or showering. As much as we might like to, we can't leave our bodies behind in cases of goo. The real world exists for a reason, and if we miss out on this, we miss out on the entire human experience of being alive. The virtual world cannot give us the fundamental requirements we need to be truly content, such as having genuinely meaningful in-person connections with other people.

We aren't born with social media accounts or a virtual watch around our wrists for a reason: we don't need them to exist. We are not products – we are people.

Illnesses

Unfortunately, it's easy to become so disconnected from our human needs, that we can easily experience challenges with our general wellbeing, that can quickly result in serious illnesses requiring medical support.

Some of these might include the below mental health issues, which can be seriously debilitating conditions. I STRONGLY advise speaking to a doctor as soon as possible if you are suffering with any of these:

- **Depression**

Feelings of hopelessness and sadness that last several days can amount to depression. Many people who use social media compulsively can experience this due to having low self-worth, low self-esteem, and low enjoyment of life, especially if they don't have a strong identity outside of the virtual world.

I've experienced depression throughout my life, which for me, feels like joy and happiness have been sucked out of my days. Feeling happy can feel very hard, and I struggle to motivate myself to do the things I know will help me to feel better, such as exercising. When we're on our phones, numbing ourselves to emotion and certain stimulating experiences, such as those in 'X is for X-rated', we stop feeling our full spectrum of emotions.

It can also fool us into believing this numbing sensation is 'relaxing', when it's actually exposing us to even more content and behaviours that make us unhappy. Whenever I've taken a break from social media, I've literally noticed my senses such as smell and noticing beauty around me to return – these simple pleasures return very quickly.

If you're experiencing this, I would advise you to start looking for one tiny way you can experience joy each day. For me it was eating an almond croissant, for others it's been going out for a walk, or speaking to someone they love. It doesn't have to be bubble baths worthy of a #selfcare hashtag, but the simple action of doing an activity in the real world that will allow you to enjoy your life. Spot those seconds of happiness, and follow them like an investigator. Each one is shining a pathway out of the black hole you might currently feel stuck in.

You will feel better, you will enjoy your life, and you will experience happiness. You can't possibly imagine how good your life is going to become, so please hold out for that time, and until then, be as kind to yourself as you possibly can.

- **Anxiety**

Feelings of constant worry and stress can amount to anxiety, of which there are several forms. For example, there may be anxiety about having to do certain things, be around certain people, or having panic attacks. It's uncontrollable thinking, worrying, and panicking – anxiety can feel as though your brain has gone into SOS mode, with a range of other symptoms such as tensing up certain muscles, or sweating, for example.

I've suffered from anxiety so much that it simply feels normal to me, to the extent that I actively avoid going out in the dark (which makes it difficult in the UK winter, as the sun sets at 4pm!). Social media can fuel anxiety, because it offers us an unlimited range of possible scenarios to worry about and attach our thoughts to. At the same time, it gives us a false sense of control, such as analysing the finer details of people's lives to try and figure out whether they might be upset with us, for example. I often find myself feeling a sense of relief when I see people post online, as I know they're still alive!

If we're literally equating life and death situations to this online world, it's obvious that we're all going to worry. Social media is not real life. As in 'C is for Content', what we see on there is biased and distorted. We can't process complex information through 180 character tweets, or infographics on Instagram – life is just not that simple. When we use social media as a self-soothing 'safety behaviour', it can become addictive, fuelling even more anxiety if we're unable to relax ourselves by checking our profiles, for example, keeping us trapped.

An anxiety-free life is possible, as in 'R is for Resilience'. By engaging with real life, we solve problems and overcome our fears. Our experiences make up who we are, but if we're refusing to have any because it feels safer to live through our phones, we're missing out on our lives.

I've found mindfulness to be extremely helpful for anxiety, including noticing when I'm worrying and asking myself what the worst possible case scenario could be. Most of the things we worry about, we can't change. Once we accept this, they disappear – it's only when we repeatedly try and fail to control these worries that they get worse.

- **Eating disorders**

As in 'D is for Disordered Eating', eating disorders are unsurprisingly, very common in relation to excessive social media use, with rates skyrocketing since Instagram became popular on a mass scale in 2012.[50] These might include anorexia, bulimia, over-exercising, bingeing and restricting, and more.

Social media can present 'healthy' information or 'inspiration' in a way that fuels negative comparisons to other people, especially in relation to their bodies, which amplifies our society's pre-existing obsession with weight. Nutritional information can easily be taken out of context to become restrictive diets, but with a veneer of justifiable reasons, such as being vegan. Veganism is great for our health and planet, but only if we cook proper food and ensure we're still getting enough nutrients. My attempt at veganism failed because I just tried to survive on bread, pasta, fruit and vegetables!

Disordered eating is so dangerous because dieting is so widely normalised in our society. Before we know it, we can easily have a full-blown eating disorder which consumes our entire lives. Having suffered with anorexia and bulimia myself, I would strongly advise addressing the root cause of these problems as soon as you notice them. Speaking from experience, sticking your head in a toilet bowl multiple times a day and spending every waking moment you have obsessing over all the food you can't eat is a horrible way to live. There is so much more to life than having a certain kind of body.

- **Body dysmorphic disorder**

---

[50] Marie Galmiche, Pierre Dechelotte, Gregory Lambert and Marie Pierre Tavolacci, 'Prevalence of eating disorders over the 2000–2018 period: a systematic literature review', *The American Journal of Clinical Nutrition, Oxford Academic,* 26 April 2019. Accessed 20 February 2022. www.academic.oup.com/ajcn/article/109/5/1402/5480601

Although the perfect body simply doesn't exist, as in 'B is for Beauty', we can convince ourselves that there is something wrong with ours. This is when a person worries a lot about their appearance, especially a particular area of their body, spends a lot of time comparing their looks with other peoples', and generally obsessively try to control or 'fix' their appearance.

Along with most of the models that I've worked with, I've suffered with this throughout my career, having been heavily pressured to meet impossible measurements that literally meant nothing. Despite knowing I am objectively very thin, it's taken a huge amount of work to stop thinking of myself as 'curvy', because of this.

It's desperately sad to hate a part of your body so much that you obsess over it, and especially when it's not even apparent to other people. Social media can work as the equivalent of mean model agents, by holding completely meaningless and impossible standards over us, literally offering us airbrushed versions of ourselves every time we look at our phones.

It can be easy to become obsessed with these standards and fixate on a particular 'issue', which makes BDD even more dangerous because it's not always apparent, and could arise in 'normalised' ways. For example, Bigorexia, or 'muscle dysmorphia', can lead to a harmful and obsessive focus on muscle development, which 1 in 10 men are estimated to experience![51] Simply viewing exercising content may not be harmful in itself, but when we become obsessed with this and looking like what we see, it can easily become dangerous.

As in 'S is for Surgery', this can end up with us become addicted to potentially life-threatening medical procedures that don't make us feel any more confident – they just give us more things to 'fix'.

---

[51] Steve Hoyles, 'Bigorexia - 1 in 10 Men Suffering?', *Hoyles Fitness*, 22 September 2015. Accessed 20 February 2022. www.hoylesfitness.com/fitness-news/bigorexia-1-in-10-men-suffering/

Therapy can be very helpful to overcome this, along with avoiding things that trigger your symptoms, such as using filters! We've all been given little jelly bags to walk around this world with that nobody truly understands, so why waste our time obsessing over the dimensions of these jelly bags, instead of using them to their full potential?

- **Addictions and substance abuse**

We can be addicted to anything, including thoughts, drugs, behaviours, smoking, alcohol, social media, work and so on! Addiction is sometimes explained in the 'Four Cs':

1. Compulsion (having an irresistible or overwhelming urge / desire to do something) – *e.g feeling an overwhelming urge to check our social media feed in the morning*

2. Cravings (sensations that mimic physical needs like hunger or thirst, which generally leads to feeling anxious when the cravings to do something aren't satisfied) – *e.g if we don't check our social media in the morning, feeling increasingly physically uncomfortable and repeated thinking about it.*

3. Consequences (when someone continues to do something despite an awareness of the negative consequences it will bring) – *e.g when we know checking our social media will distract us from getting ready, making us late for our plans, and generally lead us to feeling annoyed with ourselves for being unable to wait.*

4. Control (when someone is unable to exercise any restraint when it comes to their habits – they can't stop by themselves). *e.g checking our social media accounts, no matter how hard we try not to.*

Repeated harmful behaviours, such as taking drugs, can easily spiral out of control and destroy people's lives by becoming full blown addictions. Social media normalizes this, such as the addiction of using filters, or using 'thinspiration' pictures. It can also glamorize harmful substances such as alcohol and drugs, which are highly addictive and definitely NOT glamorous or 'cool'.

If you're feeling like a behaviour is outside of your control, please don't hesitate to ask for help. No addiction is untreatable, and the first step can often be recognising that there's a problem, especially when things like drinking alcohol and dieting are so normalised by our society. There is no shame in asking for help and every reason to do so – having your life controlled by an addiction is such a terrible waste. I lost many years of my life to alcohol, and probably even more to my screens, but if I can change, so can you.

- **Self-harm**

This is when a person intentionally injures themselves, including behaviours such as cutting or burning themselves, picking at their skin, pulling their hair, and hitting themselves. Having experienced this, I know how shameful, confusing, and addictive it can feel. It can arise from a range of situations, such as attempting to control pain or emotions, or seeking help, or self-punishment.

Social media has amplified and glamorised the problem of self-harm significantly. This is particularly girls and women – the rate for those aged 16-24 in the UK who had self-harmed increased from 6.5% in 2000 to 19.7% in 2014.[52] With everything from anti-recovery 'communities' on social media encouraging this behaviour, to group sessions, and an unlimited number of posts about it, it's unsurprising that so many of us are vulnerable to this harmful content.

If you're experiencing this, please remember that it is **not your fault.** You are not a bad person. You simply need to get the help that you very rightly deserve. You are certainly not alone, as you probably

[52] Denis Campbell, 'One in five young women have self-harmed, study reveals', *the Guardian*, 4 June 2019. Accessed 20 February 2022. www.theguardian.com/society/2019/jun/04/one-in-five-young-women-have-self-harmed-study-reveals

know from the internet – but this doesn't mean that this is okay. You deserve to live in your beautiful body and enjoy it. There are ways of processing the pain you're experiencing in a healthy way.

- **Feeling suicidal**

Suicide is the act of intentionally causing one's own death, and it's the fourth leading cause of death in 15-19 year olds.[53] Feeling suicidal is obviously not good, because not only can it lead to actually acting upon this, we can torment ourselves with harmful thoughts – and your life matters so much more than I can put into words.

I've experienced this throughout my life, and I understand how dangerous and awful it is to live like this. I was absolutely terrified to tell anyone in case I was put into a mental health hospital, but also terrified of actually acting on it in case it didn't work. This was really just shame, and fear of asking for help. I realised that I didn't want to 'die' – I just couldn't bear the emotional pain that I was experiencing, and didn't know how to process or cope with.

When we feel like we can't talk about this out of fear or guilt, especially given that we might not want to scare anyone or admit that this is really how we're feeling, it builds up, because we can't process or understand it properly. If we're suffering in silence, we might be likely to go on the internet in search of someone who is in a similar position – I remember feeling like I was the only person on Earth who felt like this.

As seen in this book, the internet can take our feelings and distort them, exposing us to more of the causes that have resulted in us first feeling this way. It is very difficult, if not impossible, to process our emotions in a healthy way on social media – Instagram and TikTok is not therapy. Although it might help to see other people are experiencing similar emotions, when you're in this state you may be

---

[53] 'Suicide', *World Health Organization,* 17 June 2021. Accessed 20 February 2022. www.who.int/news-room/fact-sheets/detail/suicide

highly vulnerable to exploitation, and **you need support in real life, not the internet.**

Please, please, please speak to someone if you're feeling suicidal. Please do not hesitate to call a helpline like Samaritans (116 123), or the others listed in the resources part of this book. Please just tell someone how you're feeling, and if you don't get the help you need, try someone else. Do not give up on the help you deserve.

It took me over 15 years to speak to someone about feeling suicidal. When I did, I received the help I needed, and was diagnosed with ADHD. I haven't felt this way since, but I will always remember how painful and all consuming it was, and how I didn't believe it would ever end. I couldn't see a way out, and I very nearly died, until I finally understood that I just didn't want to live how I was living, and sought the help to make these changes that I needed.

Two years later, I was on *Lorraine* speaking about the book I'd published that week which was on the cover of *the Times*, with a full time job, stable home, and happy relationships. This was a future I couldn't have imagined, but it was there. Hold out for your future – you can't possibly imagine all of the wonderful things that are waiting to be experienced by you.

Take control of your wellbeing

Just as social media can show us dangerously negative content, this can also be dangerously positive. No person is 'happy' 100% of the time – if we were never sad, then we'd be unable to identify what happiness is. Feeling a range of emotions is the essence of being human – you have your own unique soul.

So this isn't me telling you how to 'be happy', but simply sharing some evidence of how you can improve your overall wellbeing and get the most out of your life.

1. **Connect with other people**

As in 'F is for Friendships', having good relationships are very important to help build a sense of belonging and self-worth, provide opportunities to share positive experiences, and to have emotional support and allow you to support others.

As difficult as it might feel when you're in a negative spiral, please try your best to prioritize seeing friends or family in real life, and to be truly present with them. You can also connect with people through ways such as volunteering, which is also an excellent way of putting your difficulties into perspective!

2. **Be physically active**

Exercise helps us to raise our self-esteem, set goals and achieve them, and causes chemical changes in our brains which can help to positively change our mood. Obviously, it's also good for our physical health and keeping fit and healthy overall.

It can be extremely difficult to motivate yourself to exercise, especially if you're stuck in a scrolling vortex, but you will simply never regret it, even if it's just going for a walk. The key thing is to try and find activities that you enjoy, from rollerblading to yoga, dancing to swimming – anything! Doing exercise first thing in the day (and even sleeping in your gym clothes, if you're like me) can really help ensure this becomes part of your routine.

As above, exercise can become addictive in itself, so try to find a balance with the activities you do, and ensure these are primarily for **enjoyment** rather than looking or feeling a certain way. We can't control the outcome of exercise, but we can control how we choose to experience it.

3. **Learn new skills**

This can help us to strengthen our self-confidence & raise self-esteem, find a sense of purpose, and to connect with other people. In the world of Youtube the choices can be overwhelming, but just pick one thing at a time, and make it small!

For example, you could try cooking a new recipe, or signing up for a course at a college to learn a new language. My book writing started out as blogging! If you can, try to avoid doing this through apps, because it can be so easy to start and stop new hobbies, and beat ourselves up as a result! Start with choosing just one action to try out today, with no expectation on yourself to be 'good'.

4. Give to others

As in 'K is for Kindness', when we're kind to others this can create positive feelings and a sense of reward, give us feelings of purpose and self-worth, and helps us to connect with other people.

Kindness can be anything from complimenting a stranger to listening to a friend in need, sending a gratitude letter or volunteering at the local homeless shelter. If you can, try to do this in 'real' life, rather than online, as this will feel more meaningful. The more effort we make, the more genuine pleasure and connection we will feel as a result.

5. Mindfulness

This is paying attention to the present moment, as in 'U is for Unreal'. It can involve noticing your thoughts, feelings, body, and your current environment. As we can lose touch with both ourselves and the 'real world' in the online world, mindfulness allows us to reconnect with life in a way that feels good.

Simply noticing your thoughts is the most powerful thing you can do. You don't have to meditate for hours sitting still, but simply notice the inner voice narrating your life. Do you like what you hear? Are the thoughts helpful, or are they keeping you stuck in a loop of negative emotions? Would you say them out loud, or to somebody else? Are they true?

Challenging unhelpful thoughts has been the most life changing thing I've done, because it's helped me to see how I'm believing and acting upon thoughts that are simply not true. We have thousands of thoughts every day – so take care over which ones you're listening to.

Resources

These lists are very much non-exhaustive, so if you think something needs to be added, please send me a message at www.leannemaskell.com.

Helplines to call (UK)

- **NHS**: 111 (call 999 if you feel your life is in danger)
- **Samaritans:** 116-123
- **Campaign Against Living Miserably:** 0800 58 58 58

  Webchat page:
  https://www.thecalmzone.net/help/webchat/
- **Papyrus** (for people under 35): 0800 068 41 41

  Text: 07860039967
- **Childline** (for children and young people under 19): 0800 1111
- **SOS Silence of Suicide:** 0300 1020 505

  Email: support@sossilenceofsuicide.org
- **Shout Crisis Text Line:** text 'SHOUT' to 85258
- **YoungMinds Crisis Messenger Text Line:** text 'YM' to 85258

Charities

- **Mind:** https://www.mind.org.uk
- **Mental Health Foundation:** https://www.mentalhealth.org.uk/

- **Body Dysmorphic Disorder Foundation:** https://www.bddfoundation.org
- **BEAT:**
- **Anxiety UK**: https://www.anxietyuk.org.uk/
- **Campaign Against Living Miserably** (men's mental health charity): https://www.thecalmzone.net
- **Rethink Mental Illness:** We are Rethink Mental Illness
- **No Panic:** https://nopanic.org.uk/
- **Young Minds:** https://www.youngminds.org.uk
- **The Molly Rose foundation:** https://mollyrosefoundation.org

Books

- **For body image:** 'Women Don't Owe You Pretty', Florence Given
- **For time:** 'Time and How To Spend It', James Wallman
- **For mindfulness:** 'The Power of Now', Eckhart Tolle
- **For understanding dopamine:** 'the Molecule of More', Daniel Lieberman MD, Michael Long et al.
- **For questioning your thoughts:** 'Loving What Is', Byron Katie
- **For self-esteem:** 'Self-Compassion: the proven power of being kind to yourself', Kristen Neff
- **For addiction:** 'In the Realm of Hungry Ghosts: close encounters with addiction', Gabor Mate
- **For stress and overall health:** 'When the Body Says No: the cost of hidden stress', Gabor Mate
- **For paying attention:** 'ADHD: an A to Z', by me! Or 'The Organized Mind', Daniel Levitin

- **For boundaries:** 'Set Boundaries, Find Peace', Nedra Glover Tawwab
- **For people pleasing:** 'The Disease to Please', Harriet Braiker
- **For processing emotions:** 'How to do the work', Dr Nicole LePera
- **For eating disorders:** 'The Opposite of Butterfly Hunting', Evanna Lynch
- **For social media challenges:** 'Ten Arguments For Deleting Your Social Media Accounts Right Now', Jaron Lanier
- **For insight into 'influencer' culture:** 'Mixed Feelings', Naomi Shimada & Sarah Raphael
- **For confidence:** 'Fuck Being Humble', Stef Sword-Williams
- **For dating:** 'How To Fix A Broken Heart', Guy Winch
- **For overcoming addictions to harmful content:** 'Your Brain On Porn: Internet Pornography and the Emerging Science of Addiction', Gary Wilson, Noah Church et al.

Other recommendations

- **Body Love Sketch Club**: a 'body positive & creative empowerment project' holding joyful art workshops focusing on life drawing, healing and empowerment. Their events are seriously AMAZING and some are held online: Body Love Sketch Club Events | Eventbrite
- **Music Therapy (Talia Girton):** if you're not sure about therapy, try this! Talia takes the very simple concept of having fun and playing, and helps you to process your emotions along the way. Sessions with her changed my life and helped me during incredibly difficult times - https://www.taliagirton.com

- **Energy healing (Josephine McGrail):** when my brain has just been too emotional to be able to process anything, I've found energy healing to cut through the mess and sort my body out in ways that I simply can't put into words. I can't recommend Josephine enough.

- **No Lights No Lycra:** for dancing in the dark! Sessions are held online and in person: www.nolightsnolycra.com

- **The Joyful Wild (Emily Harding):** Emily teaches yoga in the most empowering way for 'every body', and it's impossible to leave one of her classes unhappy. I find they're especially great for people who 'don't really do yoga'! She teaches in person and online: www.emilyharding.live/join-the-joyful-wild-emily-harding-yoga-on-demand

Further resources

- Center for Humane Technology
- Your Undivided Attention podcast
- The Social Dilemma (documentary)
- The Instagram Effect (BBC)
- That Feeling When podcast